YOU MAY HAVE OSTEOPOROSIS AND NOT EVEN KNOW IT!

Consider these bone-chilling facts:

- 90% of all people with osteoporosis have not been diagnosed.
- Women have a 50% chance of fracturing a bone at some time in their life due to osteoporosis.
- If you have osteoporosis, coughing, sitting down, and even hugging a loved one can cause a fracture!

MAKE SURE YOU HAVE THE INFORMATION YOU NEED TO KEEP YOUR BONES STRONG AND HEALTHY

BONE BOOSTERS is the first simple guide to getting the essential nutrients for strong bones: not just calcium, but also vitamin A, vitamin C, phosphorus, magnesium, and zinc. In these pages you will discover:

- How to determine—right now—if you are at risk
- The truth about calcium supplements—the pros and cons
- Exciting breakthroughs in the diagnosis and treatment of osteoporosis

LIVE LONGER, LIVE STRONGER WITH *BONE BOOSTERS*

Dr. Harris McIlwain is a Board-certified rheumatologist and gerontologist and has been in practice for more than twenty years. Chosen last year by *Town and Country* as one of the Top 100 Doctors in the United States, he lectures around the world and has appeared on over 1,000 television and radio shows. Among his eleven books are *Stop Osteoarthritis Now* and *The Fibromyalgia Handbook*. Debra Fulghum Bruce has authored or coauthored twenty-nine books, including *Winning with Back Pain*.

BOOK YOUR PLACE ON OUR WEBSITE AND MAKE THE READING CONNECTION!

We've created a customized website just for our very special readers, where you can get the inside scoop on everything that's going on with Zebra, Pinnacle and Kensington books.

When you come online, you'll have the exciting opportunity to:

- View covers of upcoming books
- Read sample chapters
- Learn about our future publishing schedule (listed by publication month *and author*)
- Find out when your favorite authors will be visiting a city near you
- Search for and order backlist books from our online catalog
- Check out author bios and background information
- Send e-mail to your favorite authors
- Meet the Kensington staff online
- Join us in weekly chats with authors, readers and other guests
- Get writing guidelines
- AND MUCH MORE!

Visit our website at
http://www.kensingtonbooks.com

BONE BOOSTERS

The Essential Guide to Building Strong Bones

Harris McIlwain, M.D.,
and
Debra Fulghum Bruce

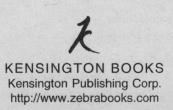

KENSINGTON BOOKS
Kensington Publishing Corp.
http://www.zebrabooks.com

KENSINGTON BOOKS are published by

Kensington Publishing Corp.
850 Third Avenue
New York, NY 10022

First Kensington Printing: May, 1998
10 9 8 7 6 5 4 3 2 1

Printed in the United States of America

Acknowledgments

While there are many who gave time for this project, including our families, we are especially appreciative of Linda McIlwain for the many hours of research she contributed to this book project. Her enthusiasm and untiring dedication were steadfast, and for this, we are indebted.

Two other women deserve acknowledgment, as well. To Denise Marcil, our literary agent, we celebrate this book with you and thank you for your commitment to osteoporosis prevention. We also are grateful for the encouragement and unfailing dedication shown by our editor, Tracy Bernstein, as she made herself available to us during the writing stages. Others who helped to make this book possible include: Brittnye Bruce, Ashley Bruce, Michael McIlwain, Jan Mashburn, M.A., and Hugh Cruse. For all of these people and their talents, we are thankful.

Abbreviations and Symbols

BBR	bone-boosting requirements	*	not available
		mcg	microgram(s)
diam.	diameter	mg	milligram(s)
fl.	fluid	oz.	ounce(s)
g	gram(s)	lb.	pound(s)
"	inches	tbsp.	tablespoon(s)
IU	international units	tsp.	teaspoon(s)
<	less than	tr.	trace

vit A = vitamin A   mag = magnesium
vit C = vitamin C   phos = phosphorus
  cal = calcium   zinc = zinc

Abbreviations and Symbols

approx.	approximately
diam.	diameter
fl.	fluid
"	inches
IU	International Units
<	less than
*	not available

THE ESSENTIAL GUIDE TO BUILDING STRONG BONES

Keeping bones strong for an entire lifetime is possible *if* you become aware of the vitamins and minerals needed to prevent osteoporosis. In listing the nutrient values of the most common foods, we used the latest information provided by the United States Department of Agriculture (**USDA**), as well as extensive data from food producers, packagers, and distributors.

When you compare this information with packaging labels or other nutrition resources, the values may differ. These variations occur for many reasons, including regional and seasonal differences in produce and how the food is gathered, processed, stored, and shipped. *Do not* let this stop you from incorporating these bone-boosting foods into your daily meal plan.

We have listed foods in the following categories:

Beverages	Milk, Cream, and Yogurt
Breads, Flour, and Grains	Miscellaneous
Candies	Nuts, Seeds, and Butters
Cereals	Pasta, Noodles, and Rice
Cheeses	Poultry
Desserts and Toppings	Prepared Foods
Eggs	Salad
Fast Foods	Salad Dressings
Fats	Seafood
Fruit	Snack Foods
Fruit Juices	Soups
Gravies, Sauces, and Dips	Soy
Meats	Vegetables

Osteoporosis is a diagnosis that more than *half* of all women over age forty-five will hear in the near future. By age seventy-five, more than *one-third* of all men have this disease. Once thought to be a consequence of aging, we now know that osteoporosis is *not* a normal progression and can be prevented.

Yet why is osteoporosis such a growing concern? Let's look at some bone-chilling facts:

- *Thirty million* Americans have osteoporosis at this time; *80 percent* are women and *less than 10 percent* are diagnosed.
- Women have a *one-in-two chance* of fracturing a bone due to osteoporosis in their lifetime—fractures that can lead to disability, disfigurement, and even death.
- A woman's risk of hip fracture is *equal* to her *combined risk* of breast, uterine, and ovarian cancer.
- *Menopause* is the single most important cause of osteoporosis due to the effect on bone of decreased levels of estrogen.
- Men are *50 percent* more likely to fracture a bone due to osteoporosis than to get prostate cancer. By age seventy-five, *one in four* men will suffer a broken hip and *one in seven* will have a spinal fracture.

The figures are startling. After osteoporosis quietly weakens your bones over the years, even normal stress on bones— such as sitting, standing, coughing, or hugging a loved one— can cause fractures that lead to chronic pain and immobility. After more fractures, osteoporosis may cause deformities, crippling, and even death.

Osteoporosis operates silently. It can start early in life and leaves no warning signs until a fracture occurs. A Washington, D.C. corporation recently gave bone density tests to all female employees and found that, among women ages forty to fifty, a startling *56 percent* had lower than normal bone density, and *19 percent* had bone density scores which indicated almost guaranteed future osteoporosis.

The good news is that osteoporosis can be prevented if you start today to *THINK BONE!* In fact, it is never too soon or too late to start keeping bones strong. With the extraordinary breakthroughs in diagnosis, prevention, and treatment of osteoporosis, almost everyone can now live fracture-free.

A simple bone density test, such as DXA (dual-energy X-ray absorptiometry), gives scientists a guaranteed way to detect this disease years *before* the first fracture occurs. This simple and inexpensive test is done in your doctor's office, and many insurance companies will cover the cost. If the test shows that your bone density is low, and you are at risk for fractures, your doctor can start you on a bone-strengthening program. This will include adding bone-boosting foods, weight-bearing and strength-training exercises, and taking bone-building medications and estrogen (for women) that actually reverse bone loss and increase bone density.

Fosamax (alendronate) is one of several new medications for use in the treatment of osteoporosis. Through numerous tests, these medications have been proven to significantly increase bone density. Over a one- to three-year period, people on this type of medication have had increases in bone density of 6 percent or more. In fact, studies show more than 90 percent of all patients respond to treatment with these medications.

Ages, Stages, and Risk Factors

Age and Bone Loss

The most critical time to build bone is during childhood and the teenage years. At this time, more bone is built than removed, so bones become larger and stronger. Recent studies reveal that 90 percent of total bone mass in females may already be in place by age sixteen. In fact, when a girl gets her first menstrual period during puberty, bone mass is increasing at its highest pace. But instead of taking advantage of building bones while the body is ''in the mood,'' the average teenage girl gets only about *300 to 800 mg* of bone-boosting calcium a day (the optimal requirement for teenage girls is *1,300–1,500 mg* a day—the equivalent of more than four glasses of milk).

If our bodies could continue to build bone throughout our lifetimes, osteoporosis would not be a problem. Yet at some point, usually in their mid-thirties, women begin to lose bone at the rate of 1 percent per year (men's bone loss usually occurs five to ten years later in life). At this time, more bone is removed than built, and osteoporosis starts throughout the skeleton. Because of hormonal changes during menopause, bone loss jumps to *about 4 percent per year* during the five to ten years after menopause (usually ages forty-five to fifty-five). Women may lose bone faster during these years than any other period. For those who didn't drink milk or eat bone-boosting foods during childhood and adolescence, or for those with several risk factors, such as cigarette smoking or lack of regular exercise, the rate is even higher.

The Stages of Osteoporosis

Understanding the stages of osteoporosis will enable you to see how bone loss and physical changes occur over time. While Stages 1 and 2 are still without any visible symptoms, it is during these stages that prevention of bone loss using the bone-boosting measures in this guide is most effective.

Stage 1 usually begins after ages thirty to thirty-five. There are no symptoms, no signs, and no detection using bone density tests. Bone removal begins to outpace bone formation.

Stage 2 usually occurs after age thirty-five. While there are no symptoms and no signs, detection is now possible using bone density tests.

Stage 3 usually occurs after age forty-five. At this stage, bones have become thin enough to result in fractures. Detection can be made using bone density tests.

Stage 4 occurs at age fifty-five and older. Not only will you have more fractures, but pain and deformity may now result. Detection is made through X-rays and bone density tests.

Are You at Risk?

There are specific genetic and environmental risk factors that set the stage for bone loss. While these factors do not cause the disease, they can alert you to an underlying problem. Some of the risk factors—such as your age, sex, race, and family history—cannot be controlled. For example, caucasian women are at higher risk than African-American women. Likewise, if your mother and grandmother had osteoporosis, your chances are greatly increased. Nonetheless, there are many factors over which you do have control, and these are the ones you can focus on changing.

—**Sex**
Women get osteoporosis about ten to fifteen years earlier than men. You cannot control this risk factor, so be sure to change the ones you can.

—**Family history**
If someone in your family has osteoporosis, especially your mother, sister, or grandmother, this places you at a much greater risk. Make important lifestyle changes for prevention.

—**Race**
If you are a Caucasian or Asian female, this places you at a higher risk for bone loss and resulting fractures. Knowing this, eliminate other risk factors.

—**Menopause or other loss of menstrual periods (amenorrhea)**

The decline of estrogen during menopause makes bone more susceptible to osteoporosis. Talk with your doctor about your specific needs, and see if supplemental estrogen may help keep your bones strong. Estrogen is still the most effective protective measure for osteoporosis after menopause. If you have abnormal loss of menstrual periods from strenuous exercise, check with your doctor to see if your exercise routine should be modified or if medications should be added.

—**Underweight and/or petite frame**

People who are underweight and who have a petite frame are at a higher risk for osteoporosis. Be sure to maintain a healthy weight, eating nutritious bone-boosting foods and exercising to keep bones strong.

—**A diet low in calcium and vitamin D**

Studies reveal that more than 90 percent of all women and 60 percent of all men get too little calcium to keep bones strong. Recently, the government has identified low calcium intake as one of the major nutritional problems in the United States today. Many people, especially women, avoid dairy products to save calories and stay slim. Some do not use dairy products because of lactose intolerance. If this applies to you, be sure you get ample calcium and vitamin D in your diet from other bone-boosting foods to be found in this guide.

—**Lack of regular exercise**

Exercise is important for building and maintaining bone mass for all ages. Make sure you exercise at least thirty minutes four to five times a week. Weight-bearing exercises, such as walking, jogging, aerobics, jumping rope, stair climbing, and dancing, stimulate bone growth. Strength training also helps to keep bones strong. Be sure to include both types of exercise in your bone-boosting program.

—**Certain medical problems**

There are some illnesses that increase your risk of getting osteoporosis. They include rheumatoid arthritis, diabetes mellitus, emphysema, chronic bronchitis, and certain types of surgery on the stomach, as well as less common medical conditions. Ask your doctor if you are at increased risk and use the bone-boosting foods and other preventative measures to stay strong.

—**Certain medications**

Some medications, such as corticosteroids (for lung diseases, allergy, and arthritis), antacids with aluminum, cholesterol-lowering drugs, heparin, and some medications used to treat prostate cancer and endometriosis can increase bone loss. Ask your doctor if your medication increases your risk of osteoporosis. See if other bone-building medications can help counteract this problem.

—**More than three cups of coffee or other caffeinated beverages daily**

Although the studies are inconclusive, high amounts of caffeine might increase the amount of calcium lost through urine. A bone-saving idea is to limit caffeine intake to two or three cups a day. Add extra milk to these drinks, or use decaffeinated beverages.

—**More than three alcoholic beverages daily**

Alcohol causes appetite suppression, resulting in decreased intakes of essential bone-boosting foods. It also impairs the absorption of calcium in the intestine. If you do drink, do so in moderation (no more than two servings a day).

—**Cigarette smoking**

Smoking doubles your risk of osteoporosis, possibly by reducing the effectiveness of the body's estrogen. Also, smokers are often underweight (another risk factor for osteoporosis). Ask your doctor about a stop-smoking program or call the American Lung Association in your community.

—**A diet high in animal protein**

Studies show that when protein consumption increases, so does calcium excretion in the urine. Excess protein binds with calcium and flushes the mineral out of the body. Limit animal protein in your diet to two small servings a day, or replace meats with soy protein or lentils.

—**A diet high in sodium**

A high salt intake can increase your loss of bone. Reduce the high-sodium processed foods in your diet to prevent possible bone loss; eat more fresh fruits and vegetables.

—**Depression**

New research shows that women who suffer one or more episodes of major depression have lower bone density, although the exact causes are not known. Be sure to seek help if you are depressed, and ask your doctor if further treatment is needed.

RATE YOUR RISK

Risk Factors You *Can't* Control	Risk Factors You *Can* Control
___Family history	___Low calcium in the diet
___Race	___Having a bone density test
___Sex	___Lack of regular exercise
___Age	___Being underweight
___Menopause	___Heavy alcohol consumption
___Certain diseases (see page 13)	___Smoking cigarettes
	___Diet high in sodium or protein
	___Certain medications (see page 13)
	Excessive exercise in athletes
	No estrogen replacement after menopause
	Caffeine consumption

SCORE OSTEOPOROSIS TEST

Take the following quiz to assess your risk for osteoporosis.

1. What is your current age? ___ years
Take this number, multiply by 3, and enter result in this space.
          ___Start

2. What is your race or ethnic group? (Check one)
African-American ___ (Enter 0)
Caucasian ___   Hispanic ___   Asian ___ (Enter 5)
Native American ___   Other ___ (Enter 5)   ___

3. Have you ever been treated for or told you have rheumatoid arthritis?
Yes ___   No ___
If yes, enter 4.   If no, enter 0.   ___

4. Since the age of 45, have you experienced a fracture (broken bone) at any of the following sites?
Hip   Yes ___   No ___   If yes, enter 4.   ___
Rib   Yes ___   No ___   If yes, enter 4.   ___
Wrist   Yes ___   No ___   If yes, enter 4.   ___

5. Do you currently take or have you ever taken estrogen? (Examples include Premarin, Estrace, Estraderm, and Estratab.)   If no, enter 1.   ___
Yes ___   No ___
Add score from questions 1 to 5.   ___**Subtotal**

6. What is your current weight?   pounds   ___
Take your weight and subtract from the **subtotal** to receive your **score.**   ___**Score**

If your final score is 6 or greater, you should be evaluated further for osteoporosis. Talk to your doctor.

Staying Fracture-free

After assessing the stages and risk factors of osteoporosis, your goal should be to stay at the stage at which the disease can be controlled. This can keep you fracture-free for your entire lifetime. Start today to prevent osteoporosis by thinking B.O.N.E.S.

- **B**oost your intake of foods that promote bone strength.

- **O**btain a bone density test from your physician.

- **N**ote the risk factors over which you have control, and make plans to change them.

- **E**xercise regularly with weight-bearing and strength-training activities.

- **S**upplement your bone-boosting plan with bone-building medications or estrogen, if warranted.

The Importance of Calcium

Calcium is the key to preventing osteoporosis. We lose a certain amount every day and must replace it through dietary measures and calcium supplements.

Studies reveal that only 10 percent of all women get adequate amounts of calcium each day. The **Bone-Boosting Requirement (BBR)** needed for osteoporosis prevention varies from *800 milligrams* a day for a preschooler to *1,500 milligrams* a day for older children, teenage girls, pregnant women, postmenopausal women not taking estrogen, and men and women sixty-five and older. The average adult between ages twenty-five and sixty-five needs at least *1,000–1,500 milligrams* per day.

More than one-third of all American households supplement their diets with calcium. Included in this statistic are the more than 50 percent of pregnant women who use calcium supplements. Yet depending on the brand, you may be getting more than you bargained for. Recent findings from the **Natural Resources Defense Council** revealed that many calcium supplements exceed the standard safe lead level of .75 microgram of lead per 1,000 milligrams of product (United States Pharmacopoeia). Lead is linked to high blood pressure, kidney problems, heart disease, and cancer. For small children and fetuses, lead can damage the central nervous system.

To stay on the safe side, try to get natural calcium through the bone-boosting foods in this book. If you use calcium supplementation, be sure to ask your doctor or pharmacist about a brand that is low in lead. When taking calcium supplements, think B.O.N.E.S. for best absorption:

- **B**e sure to take *no more* than 500 mg of supplemental calcium at one time.

- **O**nly take supplements with food for best absorption.

- **N**ever take supplements with iron, as calcium binds with iron and limits absorption.

- **E**xtra calcium taken before bedtime will give a bone-building boost during sleep.

- **S**pace supplements throughout the day to get the most benefit.

Another reason calcium-rich foods are the best source of calcium to keep bones strong is that foods offer myriad beneficial nutrients that supplements don't. A study in the *American Journal of Nutrition* reported on two groups of postmenopausal women who added to their diets either dry milk powder or calcium tablets. While both groups boosted calcium intake, because of milk's other nutrients, the women taking milk powder significantly boosted their intake of bone-boosting magnesium and zinc. Those taking calcium supplements did not.

BONE-BOOSTING REQUIREMENTS (BBR)

Children and Young Adults	Amount Per Day
0–12 months	210–270 mg
1–3 years	500 mg
4–8 years	800 mg
9–18 years	1,300–1,500 mg

Adult Women	
Pregnant and Lactating	1,000–1,300 mg
19–50 (premenopausal)	1,000 mg
51–64 (without estrogen)	1,500 mg
51–64 (with estrogen)	1,200 mg
65+ (with or without estrogen)	1,500 mg

Adult Men	
19–64	1,000 mg
65+	1,500 mg

Other Bone-Building Nutrients

While research on osteoporosis continues to point to a diet high in calcium as vital for bone strength, scientists have also identified the following bone-building nutrients to keep bones strong and help you stay fracture-free:

- **Vitamin A**—a *bone booster* necessary for normal bone growth and development. The **BBR** is 6,000 international units.

- **Vitamin C**—a *bone booster* necessary for the synthesis of collagen, a major component of bone. The **BBR** is 500 to 1,000 milligrams a day.

- **Vitamin D**—a *bone booster* that helps keep the right level of calcium and phosphorus in the bloodstream. When the body is low in vitamin D, the blood levels of calcium drop. While vitamin D is found in foods, most of this vitamin comes from sunshine. Going out-of-doors for fifteen to twenty minutes daily is a great way to boost vitamin D in the body. Yet, there are certain factors that hinder absorption, such as:

  - wearing sunscreen out-of-doors
  - aging
  - working in an office during daytime hours
  - getting sunshine through windowpane glass
  - change of seasons
  - latitude
  - time of day

When the blood levels of calcium and phosphorus drop, where does the body turn for more of these minerals? You guessed it—your bones.

New research from Tufts University suggests that postmenopausal women need 400 international units a day of vitamin D for protection against osteoporosis. Research at Boston University reveals that osteoarthritis of the knee, a common problem associated with aging, progresses more slowly in seniors who consume at least 386 international units a day, compared with those who consumed the RDA (200 international units). These studies demonstrate that many older adults would benefit from supplementation. The **BBR is** 400 to 800 international units.

- **Vitamin K**—a newly identified *bone booster!* Research shows that vitamin K is essential in promoting the laying down of calcium and preventing osteoporosis. The **BBR** is 200 micrograms (mcg) for men and women.

- **Boron**—a *bone booster* that may increase estrogen levels in the blood and help women who take estrogen replacement therapy (ERT) to retain calcium and magnesium. You should get your **BBR** of 3 milligrams a day through a diet high in fresh fruits and vegetables.

- **Fluoride**—a *bone booster* that accumulates in new bone formation sites, resulting in a net gain in bone mass. The **BBR** is 1.5 to 4 milligrams.

- **Magnesium**—a *bone booster* that regulates active calcium transport and helps to prevent fractures. Sixty percent of dietary magnesium is stored in the bone. The **BBR** is 500 to 700 milligrams per day.

- **Manganese**—a *bone booster* and antioxidant involved in bone and connective tissue development. Some researchers feel that this trace mineral may be as important as calcium in building bone! The **BBR** is between 20 and 25 milligrams daily.

- **Phosphorus**—a *bone booster* that works side by side with calcium to build strong bones and teeth. In fact, approximately 85 percent of the phosphorous in the body is found in the bones. The **BBR** is 1000 milligrams.

- **Zinc**—a *bone booster* important in the normal bone growth of children. It is part of the structure of bones, and is necessary for bones to rebuild. The **BBR** is 25 milligrams daily.

Supplement, **Not** *Substitute*

The recommended dietary allowances (RDAs) are the levels of nutrients thought to be adequate to meet the known nutrient needs of most healthy people. While the RDAs will help to prevent deficiency-related diseases such as beriberi or scurvy, there is groundbreaking scientific evidence that indicates certain nutrients should be ingested for disease prevention. In other words, the RDAs have not kept up with the medical breakthroughs.

Choosing a variety of healthful foods from this book will ensure that you are getting the proper nutrients needed to prevent osteoporosis. Of course, if your eating habits are poor, you may need supplementation with a multiple vitamin. Talk with a registered, licensed dietitian about your specific needs.

A New Superstar

Soybeans have played an essential role in Asian cultures for centuries. Heart disease, breast cancer, prostate cancer, and osteoporosis rates for Asian men and women are much lower than for Americans. Japanese women have half the rate of hip fracture of American women. Scientists attribute this to the high levels of phytoestrogens (plant estrogens) from eating a diet rich in soy.

The special isoflavones are compounds found in soy that are converted into phytoestrogens in the body. These plant ingredients mimic the hormone estrogen, but without the harmful side effects. Isoflavones appear to relieve menopausal symptoms that frequently occur because of plummeting estrogen levels during menopause. New studies have found that postmenopausal women with high concentrations of soy in their diet have stronger bones. These results indicate significant increases in both bone mineral content and bone density in the lumbar spine for women with a high soy diet. Not only is bone density increased with soy, but bone quality is improved as well. Studies show that soy protein isolate can also effectively prevent the ovarian-hormone-deficiency-associated rise in serum cholesterol.

Over the past decade, more than 2,000 new soy products

have been introduced to American consumers, including meatless pepperoni, salami, hot dogs, bacon, puddings, and dairy alternatives. Calcium-rich soy foods include calcium-set tofu, fortified soy milk, textured vegetable protein, and soy nuts. While there is no set amount of isoflavones thought to help build bones, many researchers feel that one serving of soy a day can be helpful.

What Equals One Serving of Soy?

1 cup (8 ounces) soy milk
½ cup (2 to 3 ounces) tofu
½ cup rehydrated textured
    vegetable protein (TVP)

½ cup green soybeans
3-ounce soy protein
    concentrate burger

Bone-Boosting Superstars

Calcium Superstars

Blackstrap molasses
Calcium-fortified foods
Dairy products (such as
    milk, cheese, creamed
    cheese, yogurt, ice
    cream, and cottage
    cheese)
Dried figs
Greens, mustard and turnip

Okra
Orange
Salmon (canned with
    bones)
Sardines (canned with
    bones)
Tofu (processed with
    calcium sulfate)

Vitamin A Superstars

Apricot
Cantaloupe
Carrot
Greens, turnip
Kale
Liver, beef, chicken, and
    pork

Mango
Spinach
Sweet potato
Vitamin A–fortified foods

Vitamin C Superstars

Broccoli
Grapefruit
Guava
Kohlrabi
Mango

Orange
Papaya
Peppers, red and green
Strawberries
Vitamin C–fortified foods

Vitamin D Superstars

Dairy products
Eggs and egg substitutes
Herring
Liver, beef, chicken, and
   pork
Margarine

Mackerel
Salmon
Sardines
Tuna
Vitamin D–fortified foods

Vitamin K Superstars

Asparagus
Broccoli, raw
Dairy products
Eggs
Greens, collard, mustard,
   and turnip

Lentils
Liver, beef, chicken, and
   pork
Soybeans
Spinach, raw
Whole wheat products

Boron Superstars

Beans, dried
Fruit, fresh and dried
Greens, leafy
Nuts

Peas, dried
Seeds
Vegetables

Fluoride Superstars

Anchovies, with bones
Fluoridated drinking water
Milk
Salmon, with bones
Sardines, with bones
Seaweed
Tea, especially if made with
    fluoridated water
Vegetables grown in soil
    high in fluoride

Magnesium Superstars

Avocado
Banana
Dairy products
Legumes
Nuts
Parsnips
Seafood
Soybeans
Spinach
Whole grains

Manganese Superstars

Egg
Green leafy vegetables
Lentils
Meat
Nuts
Seeds
Strawberries
Sweet potatoes
Tea
Whole grains

Phosphorus Superstars

Cheddar cheese
Eggs
Fish
Grains
Legumes
Meat
Milk
Nuts
Poultry
Tofu

Zinc Superstars

Almonds
Black-eyed peas
Crab
Peanut butter
Seafood
Sunflower seeds

Meat   Tofu
Milk   Wheat germ

Getting Started

Some bone-boosting vitamins and minerals are easy to get through a variety of foods. Because the Bone-Boosting Requirement (BBR) is low for vitamin K, boron, fluoride, and manganese, look through the Superstar lists on pages 23 to 24 to make sure you are on track. For example, a small serving of broccoli, Brussels sprouts, collards, kale, or spinach gives you a day's worth of vitamin K. You can get ample vitamin D through sun exposure of fifteen to twenty minutes each day and by drinking some vitamin D–fortified milk.

Other bone-boosting foods containing such nutrients as vitamins A and C, calcium, magnesium, phosphorus, and zinc are not always included in your daily meal plan. If your diet is low in these nutrients, consider adding these, using the extensive list of foods in your **Bone-Boosting Guide.**

In the listing, you will find a wide variety of foods and beverages with their nutrient values given for commonly consumed portion sizes. Look at the suggested Bone-Boosting Requirements (BBR) on pages 18 to 21. Then using the listing of foods, make sure that you are eating the suggested requirements for these key nutrients. Foods that have small amounts of nutrients across the board should be eaten sparingly.

By combining favorite foods, you can increase their bone-boosting benefit. For example, a plain bagel is very low in the essential vitamins and minerals needed for strong bones. If you spread 1 ounce of low-fat cream cheese on top, you have boosted your vitamin A, calcium, phosphorus, and zinc intake for the day. Top the same plain bagel with two slices of low-fat American cheese, and you have met almost one-third of your daily calcium requirement, as well as having boosted your intake of vitamin A, phosphorus, and zinc.

Add one glass of calcium-enriched orange or apple juice to boost vitamin C and calcium, and complement your meal with a spinach salad, high in bone-boosting magnesium and vitamins A and K.

Because it takes about 21 days to establish a habit such as an eating pattern, use the 21-Day Bone-Boosting Diary at the end of the book to record the foods eaten, the actual amounts, and the associated nutrients.

BONE-BOOSTING VITAMINS AND MINERALS

BEVERAGES	VIT A (IU)	VIT C (mg)	CAL (mg)	MAG (mg)	PHOS (mg)	ZINC (mg)
Alcoholic						
Beer, light (12 oz.)	0	0	18	18	43	0.11
Beer, regular (12 oz.)	0	0	18	21	43	0.07
Bloody Mary (5 oz.)	508	20	10	12	21	0.13
Daiquiri (2 oz.)	2	1	2	1	4	0.04
Screwdriver (7 oz.)	134	66	15	17	30	0.09
Tom Collins (7.5 oz.)	2	4	9	2	2	0.18
Wine, table, red (3.5 oz.)	0	0	8	13	14	0.09
Wine, table, white (3.5 oz.)	0	0	9	10	14	0.07
Nonalcoholic						
Carbonated						
Club soda (12 oz.)	0	0	18	4	0	0.36
Cola (12 oz.)	0	0	11	4	44	0.04

	VIT A (IU)	VIT C (mg)	CAL (mg)	MAG (mg)	PHOS (mg)	ZINC (mg)
Cola, with aspartame (12 oz.)	0	0	14	4	32	0.28
Ginger ale (12 oz.)	0	0	11	4	0	0.18
Lemon-lime soda	0	0	7	4	0	0.18
Orange (12 oz.)	0	0	19	4	4	0.37
Root beer (12 oz.)	0	0	19	4	0	0.26
Tonic water (12 oz.)	0	0	4	0	0	0.37

Noncarbonated

	VIT A (IU)	VIT C (mg)	CAL (mg)	MAG (mg)	PHOS (mg)	ZINC (mg)
Carob-flavor beverage mix, powder, prepared with milk (1 cup)	307	2	292	33	228	0.92
Chocolate-flavor beverage mix, powder, prepared with milk (1 cup)	311	2	301	53	255	1.28
Cocoa mix, with aspartame, powder, with added calcium, phosphorous, Swiss Miss, 1 envelope (.53 oz.)	240	0	216	31	245	0.52
Cocoa mix, with aspartame, powder, with added calcium, phosphorous, 1 packet (.675 oz.)	306	0	275	40	311	0.66
Cocoa mix, Nestlé, Carnation Hot Cocoa Mix with Marshmallows (28.0 g)	0	0	41	16	58	0.20

	VIT A (IU)	VIT C (mg)	CAL (mg)	MAG (mg)	PHOS (mg)	ZINC (mg)
Cocoa mix, Nestlé, Carnation No Sugar Added Hot Cocoa Mix (15.0 g)	0	0	123	27	135	0.60
Cocoa mix, Nestlé, Carnation Rich Chocolate Hot Cocoa Mix (28.0 g)	0	0	40	27	71	0.36
Coffee, instant, decaffeinated, powder, prepared with water (6 oz.)	0	0	5	7	5	0.05
Coffee, instant, regular, prepared with water (6 oz.)	0	0	5	7	5	0.05
Coffee, brewed, prepared with water (1 cup)	0	0	5	12	2	0.05
Fruit drink, frozen, prepared, McClain Citrus (100% vitamin C)						
Apple Melon (1 cup)	*	60	*	*	*	*
Kiwi Raspberry (1 cup)	*	60	*	*	*	*
Strawberry Lemon (1 cup)	*	60	*	*	*	*
Wild Berry Punch (1 cup)	*	60	*	*	*	*
Fruit punch drink, canned (1 cup)	35	73	20	5	2	0.30
Fruit punch-flavored drink, powder, prepared with water (1 cup)	0	31	42	3	52	0.08
Fruit punch drink, frozen concentrate, prepared with water (1 cup)	27	108	10	5	2	0.10

	VIT A (IU)	VIT C (mg)	CAL (mg)	MAG (mg)	PHOS (mg)	ZINC (mg)
Gelatin, drink, orange-flavor, powder, prepared (1 packet)	0	50	3	1	0	0.03
Lemonade-flavor drink, powder, prepared with water (1 cup)	0	34	29	3	3	0.08
Lemonade, frozen concentrate, pink, prepared with water (1 cup)	5	10	7	5	5	0.10
Lemonade, with aspartame, powder, prepared with water (1 cup)	0	6	50	2	24	0.07
Lemonade, powder, prepared with water (1 cup)	0	8	71	3	34	0.11
Malt beverage (1 cup)	5	1	12	17	52	0.05
Milk, chocolate beverage, hot cocoa, homemade (1 cup)	515	3	315	70	293	1.48
Nautilus Essentials, Soy and Milk Protein Isolate (1 packet)	5000	90	500	105	350	4.4
Nautilus Pro Drink, Milk Protein Isolate (1 packet)	2500	90	600	190	500	8
Nutri Joint, Knox unflavored gelatin drink mix, dietary supplement (1 scoop)	*	60	150	*	*	*

	VIT A (IU)	VIT C (mg)	CAL (mg)	MAG (mg)	PHOS (mg)	ZINC (mg)
Orange drink, breakfast type with juice and pulp, frozen, concentrate, prepared with water (8 oz.)	15	138	293	28	83	0.13
Orange drink, breakfast type, powder, prepared with water (1 cup)	1835	121	62	2	37	0.10
Rice Beverage, Imagine Food Rice Dream, canned (1 cup)	5	1	20	10	34	0.25
Smoothie Mix, Fountain of Youth, vanilla yogurt and protein mix, NV/Nu Vigor, dry (1.62 oz.)	5000	60	1000	*	300	13
Strawberry-flavor beverage mix, powder, prepared with milk (1 cup)	309	2	293	32	229	0.93
Tea, brewed, prepared with tap water (1 cup)	0	0	0	7	2	0.05
Tea, instant, unsweetened, powder, prepared (1 cup)	0	0	5	5	2	0.07
Tea, instant, unsweetened, lemon-flavored powder, prepared (1 cup)	0	0	5	5	2	0.07
Tea, herb, other than chamomile, brewed (1 cup)	0	0	4	2	0	0.07

	VIT A (IU)	VIT C (mg)	CAL (mg)	MAG (mg)	PHOS (mg)	ZINC (mg)
Tea, herb, chamomile, brewed (1 cup)	47	0	5	2	0	0.10
Water, bottled, Perrier, unflavored (1 cup)	0	0	33	0	0	0.00
Water, municipal (1 cup)	0	0	5	2	0	0.07

BREADS, FLOUR, AND GRAINS

Breads

Assorted

	VIT A (IU)	VIT C (mg)	CAL (mg)	MAG (mg)	PHOS (mg)	ZINC (mg)
Banana, prepared (1 slice)	278	1	13	8	35	0.21
Boston brown, canned (1 slice)	39	0	32	28	50	0.23
Cornbread						
Dry mix (1 oz.)	33	0	16	7	139	0.16
Prepared with 2% milk (1 piece)	180	0	162	16	110	0.39
Prepared with whole milk (1 piece)	158	0	161	16	109	0.38
Cracked-wheat (1 slice)	0	0	11	13	38	0.31
Egg (1 slice)	30	0	37	8	42	0.32
English muffin						
Mixed-grain (1 muffin)	4	0	129	29	98	0.64
Plain, enriched with calcium (1 muffin)	0	0	98	11	75	0.40
Plain, enriched, without calcium (1 muffin)	0	0	29	11	75	0.40
Raisin-cinnamon (1 muffin)	1	0	84	9	44	0.57

	VIT A (IU)	VIT C (mg)	CAL (mg)	MAG (mg)	PHOS (mg)	ZINC (mg)
Whole-wheat (1 muffin)	0	0	175	47	186	1.06
French or Vienna (1 medium)	0	0	19	7	26	0.22
Indian fry-Navajo (5″ dia.)	0	0	210	14	141	0.45
Irish soda, prepared (1 slice)	116	0	49	14	68	0.34
Italian (1 large slice)	0	0	23	8	31	0.26
Mixed-grain (1 large slice)	0	0	29	17	56	0.41
Oat bran (1 slice)	2	0	20	9	32	0.29
Oat-bran, reduced-calorie (1 slice)	0	0	13	11	28	0.23
Oatmeal (1 slice)	4	0	18	10	34	0.28
Phyllo dough (1 sheet)	0	0	2	3	14	0.09
Pita, white, enriched (1 large)	0	0	52	16	58	0.50
Pita, whole-wheat (1 large pita)	0	0	10	44	115	0.97
Popovers (1 popover)	117	0	38	7	56	0.30
Protein, includes gluten (1 slice)	0	0	24	10	33	0.20
Pumpernickel (1 regular slice)	0	0	18	14	46	0.39
Pumpkin, prepared (1 slice)	3259	1	11	8	32	0.20
Special formula, high-calcium, light (1 slice)	1	0	130	7	15	0.19
Special formula, high-calcium, dark (1 slice)	1	0	139	12	29	0.27
Raisin, enriched (1 slice)	1	0	17	7	28	0.19
Rye (1 slice)	1	0	23	13	40	0.37

	VIT A (IU)	VIT C (mg)	CAL (mg)	MAG (mg)	PHOS (mg)	ZINC (mg)
Tortillas, ready to bake or fry, corn (1 med., 6″)	63	0	46	17	82	0.24
Wheat (1 slice)	0	0	26	12	38	0.26
Wheat, reduced-calorie (1 slice)	0	0	18	6	21	0.19
Wheat, whole (1 slice)	0	0	20	24	64	0.54
Wheat bran (1 slice)	0	0	27	29	67	0.49
Wheat germ (1 slice)	0	0	25	10	45	0.38
White, prepared with whole milk (1 slice)	19	0	21	7	44	0.24
White, reduced-calorie (1 slice)	1	0	22	6	31	0.31

Bagels

	VIT A (IU)	VIT C (mg)	CAL (mg)	MAG (mg)	PHOS (mg)	ZINC (mg)
Cinnamon raisin (4″ dia.)	65	1	17	19	69	0.67
Egg (4″ dia.)	97	1	12	22	75	0.69
Oat bran (4½″ dia.)	4	0	13	63	182	2.29
Plain (4″ dia.)	0	0	66	26	85	0.79
Roman Meal Original (1 piece)	0	0	*	*	*	*

Biscuits

	VIT A (IU)	VIT C (mg)	CAL (mg)	MAG (mg)	PHOS (mg)	ZINC (mg)
Buttermilk (4″ dia., prepared)	83	0	237	18	166	0.55
Plain (4″ dia., prepared)	83	0	237	18	166	0.55
Mixed grain, refrigerated dough (3″ dia.)	0	0	8	14	158	0.30
Plain or buttermilk, refrigerated dough (2¼″ dia.)	0	0	4	4	98	0.10

	VIT A (IU)	VIT C (mg)	CAL (mg)	MAG (mg)	PHOS (mg)	ZINC (mg)
Bread products						
Bread crumbs, dry, grated (1 cup)	1	0	245	50	159	1.32
Bread crumbs, seasoned (1 cup)	17	0	119	46	160	1.09
Bread sticks, plain (1 stick)	0	0	2	3	12	0.09
Bread stuffing, bread, dry (1 oz.)	0	0	28	11	40	0.26
Bread stuffing, cornbread, dry (1 oz.)	45	1	22	12	32	0.21
Croutons, plain (½ oz.)	0	0	11	4	16	0.13
Croutons, seasoned (½ oz.)	3	0	14	6	20	0.13
Breakfast Breads						
French toast						
Prepared with 2% milk (1 slice)	315	0	65	11	76	0.44
Prepared with whole milk (1 slice)	298	0	64	11	76	0.44
Pancakes						
Frozen, with buttermilk (1 6″ pancake)	73	0	45	10	272	0.48
Plain, dry mix, including buttermilk (1 oz.)	19	0	68	10	184	0.20
Plain, dry mix, complete, prepared (1 6″ pancake)	25	0	97	15	257	0.30

	VIT A (IU)	VIT C (mg)	CAL (mg)	MAG (mg)	PHOS (mg)	ZINC (mg)
Pancakes, prepared from recipe						
Blueberry (6″)	153	2	159	12	116	0.42
Buckwheat (6″)	162	0	179	39	285	0.82
Buttermilk (6″)	81	0	121	12	107	0.48
Dry mix, prepared (7″)	68	0	93	15	252	0.35
Whole-wheat (6″)	292	1	323	59	481	1.34
Waffles						
Plain, dry mix, prepared (1 4″ square)	67	0	93	15	252	0.35
Plain, frozen, with buttermilk (1 4″ square)	448	0	77	7	140	0.19
Plain, prepared from recipe (7″)	171	0	191	14	143	0.51
Toaster pastry, fruit (1 Pop Tart)	501	0	14	9	58	0.34
Breakfast bar (1 bar)						
Chocolate chip (Carnation)	*	*	20	60	60	3
Chocolate crunch (Carnation)	*	*	20	60	60	3
Peanut butter w/ chocolate chips (Carnation)	*	*	20	60	60	3
Chocolate crunch, w/ chocolate chips (Carnation)	*	*	20	60	60	3

Crackers

	VIT A (IU)	VIT C (mg)	CAL (mg)	MAG (mg)	PHOS (mg)	ZINC (mg)
Cheese (1 Goldfish)	1	0	1	0	1	0.01
Cheese (1 Twig)	3	0	3	1	4	0.02
Cheese, low-sodium (1 Goldfish)	1	0	1	0	1	0.01

	VIT A (IU)	VIT C (mg)	CAL (mg)	MAG (mg)	PHOS (mg)	ZINC (mg)
Cheese, Cheez-its (1 cup)	100	0	94	22	135	0.70
Flatbread (1 cracker)	0	0	2	5	16	0.14
Matzo						
Egg (1 cracker)	12	0	11	7	45	0.21
Plain (1 cracker)	0	0	4	7	25	0.19
Whole-wheat (1 cracker)	0	0	7	38	86	0.09
Whole-wheat, low-salt (1 cracker)	0	0	2	4	12	0.09
Melba Toast (1 cracker)	0	0	3	2	6	0.06
Melba Toast, wheat (1 cracker)	0	0	2	3	8	0.08
Milk (1 cracker)	4	0	19	2	33	0.07
Oyster (1 cracker)	0	0	7	2	6	0.05
Oyster (1 cup)	0	0	54	12	47	0.35
Rye, crispbread (1 cracker)	0	0	3	8	27	0.24
Rye, cheese filling (1 cracker)	1	0	16	3	24	0.05
Saltines, fat-free, low sodium (3 crackers)	0	0	3	4	17	0.14
Saltines, soda (1 cracker)	0	0	7	2	6	0.05
Sandwich, cheese filling (1 sandwich)	2	0	18	3	28	0.04
Sandwich, with peanut butter (1 sandwich)	0	0	7	4	17	0.07
Sandwich, cheese, with peanut butter (1 sandwich)	22	0	6	4	23	0.08

	VIT A (IU)	VIT C (mg)	CAL (mg)	MAG (mg)	PHOS (mg)	ZINC (mg)
Sandwich, wheat, with cheese (1 cracker)	5	0	14	4	27	0.06
Wafer (1 cracker)	0	0	8	20	67	0.60
Wheat crackers						
Euphrates (1 cracker)	0	0	2	32	9	0.06
Harvest (1 cracker)	0	0	1	2	7	0.05
Ritz (1 cracker)	0	0	1	2	7	0.05
Wheat Thins (1 cracker)	0	0	1	2	7	0.05
Triscuits (1 cracker)	0	0	0	*	100	*
Whole-wheat (1 cracker)	0	0	7	38	86	0.09

Croissants

Apple (1 med.)	154	0	17	7	33	0.59
Butter (1 med.)	307	0	21	9	60	0.43
Cheese (1 med.)	346	0	30	14	74	0.54

Muffins, prepared with 2% milk

Blueberry (1 muffin)	80	1	108	9	83	0.31
Corn (1 muffin)	137	0	148	13	101	0.35
Oat bran (1 muffin)	10	0	36	90	214	1.05
Plain (1 muffin)	80	0	114	10	87	0.32
Wheat bran (1 muffin)	478	5	107	45	163	1.57

Muffins, prepared with whole milk

Blueberry (1 muffin)	63	1	107	9	82	0.31
Corn (1 muffin)	117	0	147	13	100	0.35
Plain (1 muffin)	61	0	113	9	87	0.32
Wheat bran (1 muffin)	459	5	106	45	162	1.57

Rolls	VIT A (IU)	VIT C (mg)	CAL (mg)	MAG (mg)	PHOS (mg)	ZINC (mg)
Cinnamon, refrigerated dough (1 roll)	0	0	10	4	104	0.10
Egg (1 roll)	26	0	21	9	35	0.32
French (1 roll)	2	0	35	8	32	0.29
Oat bran (1 roll)	3	0	28	10	34	0.28
Plain (1 roll)	0	0	30	24	64	0.57
Plain, prepared with 2% milk (1 roll)	118	0	21	7	44	0.25
Plain, prepared with whole milk (1 roll)	108	0	21	7	44	0.25
Sweet rolls, prepared with raisins (1 roll)	233	0	36	16	63	0.38
Sweet rolls, prepared with cheese (1 roll)	135	0	78	13	65	0.42
Hamburger (1 roll)	0	0	60	9	38	0.27
Hamburger, mixed-grain (1 roll)	0	0	41	21	52	0.46
Hard (1 roll)	0	0	54	15	57	0.54
Hot dog (1 roll)	0	0	60	9	38	0.27
Hot dog, mixed-grain (1 roll)	0	0	41	21	52	0.46
Plain (1 roll)	129	1	43	10	46	0.35
Soft (1 roll)	0	0	30	24	63	0.57
Wheat (1 roll)	0	0	50	12	33	0.29
Whole-wheat, dinner roll (1 roll)	0	0	30	24	64	0.57
Whole-wheat, submarine (1 roll)	0	0	100	80	210	1.89

Flour						
Acorn, full fat (1 oz.)	15	0	12	31	29	0.18
Amaranth (1 cup)	0	8	298	519	887	6.2
Arrowroot (1 cup)	0	0	51	4	14	0.09

	VIT A (IU)	VIT C (mg)	CAL (mg)	MAG (mg)	PHOS (mg)	ZINC (mg)
Buckwheat, whole-groat (1 cup)	0	0	49	301	404	3.74
Carob (1 cup)	1	0	358	56	81	0.95
Corn, masa, enriched (1 cup)	0	0	161	125	254	2.02
Corn, whole-grain, yellow (1 cup)	549	0	8	109	318	2.02
Cottonseed, partially defatted (1 cup)	408	2	449	678	1501	10.99
Peanut, defatted (1 cup)	0	0	84	222	456	3.06
Peanut, low-fat (1 cup)	0	0	78	29	305	3.59
Pecan (1 oz.)	34	1	9	34	78	1.45
Potato (1 cup)	0	34	59	158	319	2.92
Rice, brown (1 cup)	0	0	17	177	533	3.87
Rice, white (1 cup)	0	0	16	55	155	1.26
Rice bran, crude (1 cup)	0	0	67	922	1979	7.13
Rye, medium (1 cup)	0	0	25	77	211	2.03
Semolina, enriched (1 cup)	0	0	28	78	227	1.75
Sesame, low-fat (1 oz.)	18	0	42	96	215	2.84
Sesame, partially defatted (1 oz.)	20	0	43	103	230	0.03
Soy, defatted (1 cup)	40	0	241	290	674	2.46
Soy, low-fat (1 cup)	35	0	165	202	522	1.04
Sunflower seed, partially defatted (1 cup)	31	1	73	221	441	3.17
Triticale, whole grain (1 cup)	0	0	46	199	417	3.46
Wheat, white, all-purpose, enriched (1 cup)	0	0	19	28	135	0.88
Wheat, white, all-purpose, enriched, calcium-fortified (1 cup)	0	0	315	28	135	0.87

	VIT A (IU)	VIT C (mg)	CAL (mg)	MAG (mg)	PHOS (mg)	ZINC (mg)
Wheat, white, cake, enriched (1 cup)	0	0	19	22	117	0.85
Wheat, white, enriched (1 cup)	0	0	21	34	133	1.17
Wheat, white, tortilla mix, enriched (1 cup)	0	0	228	23	233	0.71
Wheat, whole (1 cup)	0	0	41	166	415	3.52
Grains						
Almond meal, partially defatted, without added salt (1 oz.)	0	0	120	82	259	0.8
Amaranth, cereal grain (½ cup)	0	4	149	260	444	3.1
Amaranth, cereal grain (1 cup)	0	8	298	519	887	6.2
Barley (½ cup)	20.5	0	31	123	243	2.55
Barley (1 cup)	41	0	61	245	486	5.1
Barley, pearled, raw (½ cup)	22	0	29	79	221	2.13
Barley, pearled, raw (1 cup)	44	0	58	158	442	4.26
Bran						
Corn, crude (1 cup)	54	0	32	49	55	1.19
Oat, raw (1 cup)	0	0	55	221	670	2.92
Rice, crude (1 cup)	0	0	67	922	1979	7.13
Wheat, crude (1 cup)	0	0	42	354	588	4.22
Buckwheat groats, roasted, dry (1 cup)	0	0	28	362	523	3.7
Bulgar, cooked (½ cup)	0	0	18	58	73	1.04
Cornmeal						
Degermed, enriched, yellow (1 cup)	570	0	7	55	116	0.99
Self-rising, degermed, yellow (1 cup)	570	0	483	68	860	1.38

	VIT A (IU)	VIT C (mg)	CAL (mg)	MAG (mg)	PHOS (mg)	ZINC (mg)
Self-rising, plain, enriched, white (1 cup)	0	0	440	105	991	2.4
Self-rising, wheat flour added, enriched (1 cup)	0	0	508	91	1107	2.4
Couscous, cooked (½ cup)	0	0	14	14	39	0.46
Couscous, cooked (1 cup)	0	0	28	28	78	0.92
Millet, cooked (½ cup)	0	0	3.5	53	120	1.09
Millet, cooked (1 cup)	0	0	7	106	240	2.18
Quinoa (½ cup)	0	0	51	179	349	2.8
Quinoa (1 cup)	0	0	102	357	697	5.61
Rice						
Brown, long-grained, cooked (½ cup)	0	0	10	2	81	0.62
Brown, long-grained, cooked (1 cup)	0	0	19	4	162	1.24
White, glutinous, cooked (½ cup)	0	0	8	9	34	0.39
White, glutinous, cooked (1 cup)	0	0	16	18	68	0.78
White, long-grain, parboiled, enriched (½ cup)	0	0	17	11	37	0.27
White, long-grain, parboiled, enriched (1 cup)	0	0	33	21	74	0.54
Wild, cooked (½ cup)	0	0	3	27	68	1.1
Wild, cooked (1 cup)	0	0	5	53	135	2.2
Sesame meal, partially defatted (1 cup)	19	0	43	98	219	2.9
Semolina, enriched (1 cup)	0	0	28	79	227	1.75
Soy meal, defatted, raw (1 cup)	48	0	297	373	855	6.17

	VIT A (IU)	VIT C (mg)	CAL (mg)	MAG (mg)	PHOS (mg)	ZINC (mg)
Triticale (1 cup)	0	0	71	250	687	6.62
Wheat germ (¼ cup)	32	0	14	84	325	4.64
Wheat germ (½ cup)	64	0	28	168	650	9.28

CANDIES

	VIT A (IU)	VIT C (mg)	CAL (mg)	MAG (mg)	PHOS (mg)	ZINC (mg)
Almond Joy, 1 bar (1.76 oz.)	7	0	40	33	70	0.40
Bar None, 1 bar (1.5 oz.)	57	0	62	31	86	0.53
Cadbury's Caramello, 1 bar (1.6 oz.)	148	1	89	19	72	0.43
Caramels, chocolate-flavor roll, 1 bar (2.25 oz.)	5	0	15	20	25	0.34
Chocolate, baking, unsweetened, 1 square (1 oz.)	28	0	21	88	118	1.14
Chocolate, chips, semisweet, 60 pieces (1 oz.)	6	0	9	33	37	0.46
Chocolate, sweet, 1 bar (1.45 oz.)	8	0	10	46	60	0.62
Chocolate, with nuts, prepared, 1 piece (19.0 g)	38	0	10	9	18	0.14
Demet's Turtles, 1 piece (17.0 g)	28	0	27	9	34	0.25
Fudge						
Brown sugar, with nuts, prepared, 1 piece (14.0 g)	11	0	16	7	12	0.09
Chocolate, prepared, 1 piece (17.0 g)	32	0	7	4	10	0.07
Chocolate with nuts, prepared, 1 piece (19.0 g)	38	0	10	9	18	0.14

	VIT A (IU)	VIT C (mg)	CAL (mg)	MAG (mg)	PHOS (mg)	ZINC (mg)
Vanilla with nuts, prepared, 1 piece (15.0 g)	30	0	7	4	11	0.08
Golden Almond, 1 bar (3 oz.)	125	0	279	94	230	1.45
Golden Almond Solitaires, 1 package (3 oz.)	43	0	305	100	255	1.56
Goobers Chocolate Covered Peanuts, 1 package (1.375 oz.)	0	0	50	46	115	0.85
Gumdrops, starch jelly pieces, 10 gummy worms (74.0 g)	0	0	2	1	1	0.00
Jelly beans, 10 small (11.0 g)	0	0	0	0	0	0.01
Krackel, 1 bar (1.65 oz.)	23	0	84	26	104	0.57
M & M's Milk Chocolate Mini-Baking Bits, 1 serving (14.2 g)	32	0	16	7	24	0.15
M & M's Peanut Chocolate Candies, 1 package (1.67 oz.)	44	0	48	29	89	0.64
M & M's Plain Chocolate Candies, 1 package (1.69 oz.)	97	0	50	20	72	0.46
M & M's Semisweet Chocolate Mini-Baking Bits (1 tbsp.)	10	0	5	15	17	0.21
Milk chocolate candies, 1 bar (1.55 oz.)	81	0	84	26	95	0.61
Milk chocolate-coated peanuts, 10 pieces (40.0 g)	0	0	42	36	85	0.75
Mints, After Eight, 5 pieces (41.0 g)	8	0	9	19	23	0.24

	VIT A (IU)	VIT C (mg)	CAL (mg)	MAG (mg)	PHOS (mg)	ZINC (mg)
Mounds, 1 package (1.9 oz.)	5	0	12	37	65	0.56
Mr. Goodbar, 1 bar (1.75 oz.)	20	0	56	48	140	0.90
Oh Henry! Bar, 1 bar (2 oz.)	27	0	62	35	103	0.70
Raisinets Chocolate Covered Raisins, 1 package (1.51 cup)	17	0	49	20	65	0.36
Reese's Peanut Butter Cups, 1 package (1.6 oz.)	30	0	35	38	108	0.63
Reese's Pieces Candy, 1 package (1.95 oz.)	11	0	73	46	127	0.61
Rolo Caramels in Milk Chocolate, 1 piece (3.0 g)	2	0	4	1	5	0.02
Skør Toffee Candy Bar, 1 bar (1.4 oz.)	112	0	45	14	60	0.30
Snickers Bar, 1 bar (2 oz.)	87	0	54	39	105	0.81
Special Dark Sweet Chocolate Bar, Hershey, 1 bar (1.45 oz)	8	0	8	47	66	0.62
Symphony Milk Chocolate Bar, 1 bar (1.4 oz.)	28	0	94	22	100	0.45
Twix Caramel Cookie Bars, 1 package (2.06 oz.)	55	0	52	19	70	0.45
Twix Peanut Butter Cookie Bar, 1 package, 2 bars (1.89 oz.)	39	0	42	40	103	0.76

	VIT A (IU)	VIT C (mg)	CAL (mg)	MAG (mg)	PHOS (mg)	ZINC (mg)
Twizzlers, Strawberry Candy (5 oz. package)	0	0	50	9	440	0.23
Yogurt, confectioner's coating candy (50 g edible portion)	18	0	100	6	88	0.37
York Peppermint Pattie, 1 large patty (43.0 g)	2	0	7	27	41	0.33

CEREALS

Hot, Measured, uncooked

	VIT A (IU)	VIT C (mg)	CAL (mg)	MAG (mg)	PHOS (mg)	ZINC (mg)
Corn grits, instant, plain, Quaker (1 packet)	0	0	6	10	31	0.19
Corn grits, yellow, enriched, dry (1 tbsp.)	43	0	0	3	7	0.04
Cream of Rice (¼ cup)	0	0	10	10	54	0.48
Cream of Rice (½ cup)	0	0	20	20	108	0.96
Cream of Wheat, mix'n eat, plain (1 packet)	1250	0	20	8	20	0.24
Cream of Wheat, instant (2 tbsp.)	0	0	32	8	24	0.22
Cream of Wheat, regular (2 tbsp.)	0	0	30	6	24	0.18
Malt-O-Meal, plain (2 tbsp.)	0	0	3	3	15	0.10
Mother's Oat Bran (½ cup)	40	0	32	96	278	1.68
Oatmeal, MultiGrain, Quaker (½ cup)	3	0	14	46	138	1.28
Oatmeal, instant, Power Ranger, fruit punch flavor, Quaker (1 packet)	1273	0	176	35	121	0.80

	VIT A (IU)	VIT C (mg)	CAL (mg)	MAG (mg)	PHOS (mg)	ZINC (mg)
Oatmeal, instant, Quaker, Apples and Cinnamon (1 packet)	1050	0	106	30	116	0.69
Oatmeal, instant, Quaker, Maple and Brown Sugar (1 packet)	1008	0	105	39	132	0.90
Roman Meal, plain (⅓ cup)	0	0	20	74	146	1.21
Wheatena (¼ cup)	0	0	10	46	134	1.54

Ready to Eat

	VIT A (IU)	VIT C (mg)	CAL (mg)	MAG (mg)	PHOS (mg)	ZINC (mg)
All-Bran (½ cup)	750	15	106	129	294	3.75
All-Bran with extra fiber (½ cup)	866	17	116	120	287	4.32
Basic 4 (1 cup)	1250	15	310	40	232	3.75
Berry Berry Kix (¾ cup)	750	15	66	6	37	3.75
Boo Berry (1 cup)	0	15	20	3	31	3.75
Bran, 100% (1 cup)	0	63	46	312	801	5.74
Bran Buds (⅓ cup)	750	15	20	83	166	6.45
Bran Chex (1 cup)	107	26	29	69	173	6.48
Bran Flakes, 40%, Ralston Purina (1 cup)	2160	26	23	118	273	2.04
Cap'n Crunch (¾ cup)	36	0	5	10	29	3.75
Cheerios (1 cup)	1250	15	55	33	114	3.75
Apple Cinnamon (¾ cup)	750	15	35	20	65	3.75
Honey Nut (1 cup)	750	15	20	29	103	3.75
Multigrain (1 cup)	750	15	57	30	114	3.75
Cinnamon Toast (¾ cup)	750	15	42	14	74	3.75
Clusters (1 cup)	0	9	72	52	153	1.05
Cocoa Krispies (¾ cup)	750	15	4	11	29	1.49

	VIT A (IU)	VIT C (mg)	CAL (mg)	MAG (mg)	PHOS (mg)	ZINC (mg)
Cocoa Pebbles (1 cup)	1411	0	6	13	25	1.70
Cocoa Puffs (1 cup)	0	15	33	7	43	3.75
Common Sense (¾ cup)	750	0	15	48	153	3.75
Complete Bran Flakes (¾ cup)	1208	15	14	60	150	3.75
Corn Chex (1 cup)	146	15	3	4	11	0.10
Corn Flakes, Kellogg (1 cup)	700	14	1	3	11	0.17
Corn Flakes, Ralston Purina (1 cup)	95	0	2	3	10	0.06
Corn Pops (1 cup)	775	16	3	3	7	1.55
Count Chocula (1 cup)	0	15	29	9	41	3.75
Country Corn Flakes (1 cup)	750	15	53	7	39	3.75
Cracklin' Oat Bran (¾ cup)	842	17	25	77	187	1.65
Crispix (1 cup)	750	15	4	7	27	1.51
Crispy Wheaties 'N Raisins (1 cup)	1250	0	69	42	140	1.08
Crunchy Bran (¾ cup)	38	0	21	14	36	3.75
Fiber One (½ cup)	0	9	59	68	168	1.24
Frankenberry (1 cup)	0	15	25	3	28	3.75
Froot Loops (1 cup)	703	14	3	9	21	3.75
Frosted Bran (¾ cup)	726	15	9	38	92	3.63
Frosted Flakes (¾ cup)	775	16	1	3	8	0.16
Fruity Pebbles (1 cup)	1411	0	4	9	19	1.70
Golden Grahams (¾ cup)	750	15	14	9	36	3.75
Granola, homemade (1 cup)	45	2	99	217	564	4.95
Granola, Low-Fat, Kellogg (½ cup)	842	0	23	47	135	4.24
Granola, Low-Fat with Raisins, Kellogg (⅔ cup)	688	0	24	46	127	3.47

	VIT A (IU)	VIT C (mg)	CAL (mg)	MAG (mg)	PHOS (mg)	ZINC (mg)
Grape-Nuts (½ cup)	2403	0	5	37	137	1.20
Grape-Nuts Flakes (1 oz.)	1250	0	11	31	84	0.57
Healthy Choice Multi-Grain Flakes (1 cup)	500	0	9	29	86	1.50
Heartland Natural Cereal, Plain (1 cup)	64	1	75	147	416	3.04
Heartland Natural Cereal with Coconut (1 cup)	57	1	66	138	380	2.74
Heartland Natural Cereal with Raisins (1 cup)	63	1	66	141	377	2.83
Honey Bran (1 cup)	1543	19	16	46	132	0.90
Just Right (1 cup)	1250	0	14	34	106	0.88
Just Right Fruit & Nut (1 cup)	1146	0	0	33	109	1.05
Kaboom (1¼ cup)	750	15	50	19	88	3.75
King Vitaman (1½ cup)	1044	12	4	26	79	3.91
Life, Cinnamon (1 cup)	16	0	135	42	181	6.29
Life (¾ cup)	12	0	98	31	136	4.00
Maltex (¼ cup)	0	0	14	42	133	1.38
Mueslix Apple & Almond Crunch (¾ cup)	778	0	34	63	175	3.14
Mueslix Raisin & Almond Crunch, with Dates (⅔ cup)	200	0	20	47	133	3.74
Natural Bran Flakes, Post (1 cup)	2072	0	21	102	296	2.49
Natural Cereal, 100%, with Apple and Cinnamon, Quaker (1 oz.)	16	0	43	20	96	0.54
Natural Cereal, 100%, with Oats and Honey, Quaker (½ cup)	3	0	46	50	149	1.15

	VIT A (IU)	VIT C (mg)	CAL (mg)	MAG (mg)	PHOS (mg)	ZINC (mg)
Natural Cereal, 100% with Oats, Honey, and Raisins, Quaker (½ cup)	4	0	39	48	150	1.08
Natural Cereal, 100% with Raisins and Dates, Quaker (1 oz.)	16	0	41	32	90	0.54
Nature Valley, Cinnamon & Raisins Granola (¾ cup)	0	0	43	55	160	0.91
Nature Valley Low-Fat Fruit Granola (⅔ cup)	0	0	40	19	180	0.88
Nut & Honey Crunch (1¼ cup)	750	15	6	5	36	0.39
Nutri-Grain, Almond and Raisin (30 g)	0	0	102	8	113	2.4
Nutri-Grain, Wheat (¾ cup)	0	15	10	24	108	3.75
Nuttlettes (½ cup)	*	*	160	*	*	*
Oat Flakes, Post (1 cup)	2116	0	68	58	176	2.54
Oatmeal Crisp with Almonds (1 cup)	0	9	36	57	144	3.75
Oatmeal Squares, Quaker (1 cup)	563	7	36	70	186	4.22
Product 19 (1 cup)	750	60	3	12	40	15.00
Puffed Rice, Quaker (1 cup)	0	0	1	4	17	0.15
Puffed Wheat, Quaker (1¼ cup)	2	0	4	20	50	0.46
Raisin Bran, Kellogg (1 cup)	832	0	40	89	214	4.15
Raisin Bran, Post (1 cup)	2469	0	26	95	235	2.97
Raisin Bran, Ralston Purina (1 cup)	1852	2	27	85	248	1.67

	VIT A (IU)	VIT C (mg)	CAL (mg)	MAG (mg)	PHOS (mg)	ZINC (mg)
Raisin Nut Bran, General Mills (1 cup)	0	0	74	54	163	1.11
Raisin Squares, Kellogg (¾ cup)	0	0	19	48	160	1.54
Rice Chex (1 cup)	20	18	5	8	32	0.46
Rice Krispies (1¼ cup)	825	17	3	16	44	0.60
Rice Krispies, Apple-Cinnamon (¾ cup)	776	16	2	8	25	0.33
Rice Krispies Treats Cereal (¾ cup)	750	15	2	6	20	0.30
S'mores Grahams (¾ cup)	750	15	14	11	41	3.75
Shredded wheat, large biscuit (1 oblong biscuit)	0	0	10	43	91	0.63
Shredded wheat, small biscuit (1 cup)	0	0	9	33	88	0.82
Special K (1 cup)	750	15	5	18	51	3.75
Strawberry Squares (1 cup)	0	0	22	66	169	1.65
Sugar Frosted Flakes, Ralston (1 cup)	1675	20	4	3	10	0.82
Sun Country Granola, Raisin and Date (½ cup)	0	0	24	26	92	0.50
Super Sugar Crisp (1 cup)	1455	0	7	20	44	1.75
Team (1 cup)	1852	22	6	12	65	0.58
Toasted Brown Sugar Squares, Healthy Choice (1¼ cup)	509	0	19	59	194	1.54
Total (¾ cup)	1250	60	258	32	211	15.00
Total Corn Flakes (1⅓ cup)	1250	60	237	8	110	15.00

	VIT A (IU)	VIT C (mg)	CAL (mg)	MAG (mg)	PHOS (mg)	ZINC (mg)
Total Raisin Bran (1 cup)	1250	0	238	45	259	14.00
Tripples (1 cup)	1250	15	41	7	35	3.75
Uncle Sam, Low-Sodium (1 cup)	*	1	40	*	*	*
Wheat Chex (1 cup)	0	24	18	58	182	1.23
Wheat germ, toasted, plain (1 oz.)	0	2	13	91	325	4.72
Wheat germ, Kretchmer Honey Crunch (1⅔ tbsp.)	13	0	7	38	142	1.94
Wheaties (1 cup)	750	15	55	32	96	0.71

CHEESES

	VIT A (IU)	VIT C (mg)	CAL (mg)	MAG (mg)	PHOS (mg)	ZINC (mg)
American, pasteurized process, 1 slice (1 oz.)	343	0	175	6	211	0.85
Blue (1 oz.)	204	0	150	7	110	0.75
Brick (1 oz.)	307	0	191	7	128	0.74
Brie (1 oz.)	189	0	52	6	53	0.68
Camembert (1 oz.)	262	0	110	6	98	0.68
Caraway (1 oz.)	299	0	191	6	139	0.83
Cheddar (1 oz.)	300	0	205	8	145	0.88
Cheddar, low-fat (1 oz.)	66	0	118	5	137	0.52
Cheddar, low sodium (1 oz.)	297	0	200	8	137	0.88
Cheshire (1 oz.)	279	0	182	6	131	0.79
Colby (1 oz.)	293	0	194	7	129	0.87
Colby, low-fat (1 oz.)	66	0	118	5	137	0.52
Cottage cheese						
Calcium enriched, 1% fat (½ cup)	0	0	200	*	*	*
Creamed, large curd, not packed (1 cup)	367	0	135	12	297	0.83

	VIT A (IU)	VIT C (mg)	CAL (mg)	MAG (mg)	PHOS (mg)	ZINC (mg)
Creamed, small curd, not packed (1 cup)	367	0	135	12	297	0.83
Creamed, with fruit, not packed (1 cup)	278	0	108	9	236	0.66
Lactose-reduced, 1% fat (½ cup)	0	0	100	*	*	*
1% fat, not packed (1 cup)	84	0	138	12	302	0.86
2% fat, not packed (1 cup)	158	0	155	14	340	0.95
Uncreamed, dry, large or small curd, not packed (1 cup)	44	0	46	6	151	0.68
Cream cheese (1 oz.)	405	0	23	2	30	0.15
Cream cheese, fat-free (100 g)	930	0	185	14	434	0.88
Edam (1 oz.)	260	0	207	8	152	1.06
Feta (1 oz.)	127	0	140	5	96	0.82
Fontina (1 oz.)	333	0	156	4	98	0.99
Fondue, cheese (½ cup)	447	0	514	25	331	2.12
Gjetost (1 oz.)	316	0	113	20	126	0.32
Goat, hard type (1 oz.)	451	0	254	15	207	0.45
Goat, semisoft type (1 oz.)	378	0	85	8	106	0.19
Goat, soft (1 oz.)	378	0	40	4	73	0.26
Gouda (1 oz.)	183	0	198	8	155	1.11
Gruyère (1 oz.)	346	0	287	10	172	1.11
Limburger (1 oz.)	363	0	141	6	112	0.6
Monterey (1 oz.)	269	0	212	8	126	0.85
Mozzarella						
Part skim (1 oz.)	166	0	183	7	131	0.78

	VIT A (IU)	VIT C (mg)	CAL (mg)	MAG (mg)	PHOS (mg)	ZINC (mg)
Part skim, low-moisture (1 oz.)	178	0	207	8	149	0.89
Whole milk (1 oz.)	225	0	147	5	105	0.63
Whole milk, low-moisture (1 oz.)	256	0	163	6	117	0.01
Muenster (1 oz.)	318	0	203	8	133	0.8
Neufchatel (1 oz.)	322	0	21	2	39	0.15
Parmesan						
Grated (1 oz.)	199	0	390	14	229	0.9
Grated (1 tbsp.)	35	0	69	3	40	0.16
Hard (1 oz.)	171	0	336	12	197	0.78
Lactose-Free, Parmesan Flavor, Grated Topping, Formagg (2 tbsp.)	0	0	60	*	*	*
Pimento, pasteurized pimento (1 oz.)	358	1	174	6	211	0.85
Port du salut (1 oz.)	378	0	184	7	102	0.74
Provolone (1 oz.)	231	0	214	8	141	0.92
Queso anejo, Mexican (1 oz.)	63	0	193	8	126	0.83
Queso asadero, Mexican (1 oz.)	63	0	188	7	126	0.86
Ricotta, part-skim milk (1 oz.)	122	0	77	4	52	0.38
Ricotta, whole milk (1/2 cup)	608	0	257	14	196	1.44
Romano (1 oz.)	162	0	302	12	216	0.73
Roquefort (1 oz.)	297	0	188	8	111	0.59
Sauce, cheese, prepared (2 tbsp.)	182	0	93	6	69	0.39
Swiss, pasteurized (1 oz.)	229	0	219	8	216	1.02
Swiss, Reduced Fat, Sargento (1 slice)	500	*	300	*	*	*
Tilsit (1 oz.)	296	0	198	4	142	0.99

DESSERTS AND TOPPINGS	VIT A (IU)	VIT C (mg)	CAL (mg)	MAG (mg)	PHOS (mg)	ZINC (mg)
Apple crisp, prepared (½ cup)	193	3	39	10	35	0.23
Brownies						
Commercially prepared (1 Little Debbie package twin)	42	0	18	19	62	0.44
Dry mix, prepared, 1 brownie (2″ square)	15	0	6	11	26	0.2
Dry mix, special dietary prepared, 1 brownie (2″ square)	0	0	3	1	11	0.03
Prepared from recipe, 1 brownie (2″ square)	184	0	14	13	32	0.23
Cakes						
Angel food Commercially prepared (1 slice)	0	0	40	3	66	0.02
Dry mix, prepared (1 piece)	0	0	42	4	116	0.07
Prepared from recipe (1 piece)	0	0	3	5	13	0.07
Boston cream pie, prepared from recipe (1 piece)	180	0	93	16	91	0.44
Carrot, dry mix, pudding-type without frosting, 1 piece (1/12 of 9″ dia.)	790	2	77	5	123	0.22

	VIT A (IU)	VIT C (mg)	CAL (mg)	MAG (mg)	PHOS (mg)	ZINC (mg)
Carrot, prepared from recipe with cream cheese frosting (1 piece)	3827	1	28	20	79	0.54
Cheesecake						
Commercially prepared (1 piece)	442	1	41	9	74	0.41
Plain, prepared from recipe with cherry topping (1 piece)	1275	1	61	10	101	0.57
Prepared from mix, no-bake type (1 piece)	362	1	170	19	232	0.46
Prepared from recipe (1 piece)	1354	1	74	10	123	0.7
Chocolate, commercially prepared with chocolate frosting (1 piece)	61	0	28	22	78	0.16
Chocolate, dry mix, pudding-type, prepared without frosting (1 piece)	81	1	64	19	146	0.49
Coffee cake						
Cheese (1 piece)	178	0	45	11	75	0.45
Cinnamon with crumb topping (1 piece)	61	0	34	14	68	0.51
Fruit (1 piece)	70	0	23	9	59	0.33
Commercially prepared (1 piece)	34	0	14	7	23	0.12
Fruitcake, prepared from recipe (1 piece)	61	4	55	29	66	0.59

	VIT A (IU)	VIT C (mg)	CAL (mg)	MAG (mg)	PHOS (mg)	ZINC (mg)
Pineapple upside-down, prepared from recipe (1/9 of 8" square)	291	1	138	15	94	0.36
Pound						
Commercially prepared, with butter (1 oz.)	172	0	10	3	39	0.13
Commercially prepared, fat-free (1 oz.)	27	0	12	3	41	0.09
Prepared from recipe, with butter (1/16 of loaf cake)	524	0	13	5	44	0.27
Shortcake, biscuit-type, prepared from recipe (1 cake, 3" dia.)	47	0	133	10	93	0.31
Sponge, prepared from recipe, 1 piece (1/12 of 16 oz. cake)	163	0	27	6	63	0.37
White						
Prepared from recipe, with coconut frosting (1 piece)	43	0	101	13	78	0.37
Prepared from recipe, without frosting (1 piece)	41	0	96	9	69	0.24
Dry mix, pudding-type, without frosting (1 piece)	0	0	35	5	123	0.12
Yellow, dry mix, pudding-type, without frosting (1 piece)	80	0	57	5	133	0.26

	VIT A (IU)	VIT C (mg)	CAL (mg)	MAG (mg)	PHOS (mg)	ZINC (mg)
Yellow, prepared from recipe, without frosting (1 piece)	95	0	99	8	80	0.31

Cookies

Animal crackers (2 oz.)	0	0	25	10	65	0.37
Arrowroot (2 oz.)	0	0	25	10	65	0.37
Butter, commercially prepared, enriched (1 cookie)	30	0	2	1	5	0.02
Chocolate chip						
Chips Ahoy, Nabisco (1 cookie)	1	0	4	4	15	0.09
Chocolate Chunk Pecan, Pepperidge Farm (1 cookie)	1	0	3	4	13	0.08
Commercially prepared, regular, lower fat (1 cookie)	0	0	2	3	8	0.07
Commercially prepared, soft, lower fat (1 cookie)	0	0	2	5	8	0.07
Refrigerated dough (1 med. cookie)	7	0	3	3	9	0.07
Rich 'n Chips, Pecan Chips, Keebler (1 large cookie)	1	0	4	4	15	0.09
Chocolate sandwich, with cream filling (1 cookie)	0	0	3	5	10	0.08
Chocolate sandwich, with extra cream (1 cookie)	0	0	3	4	12	0.09

	VIT A (IU)	VIT C (mg)	CAL (mg)	MAG (mg)	PHOS (mg)	ZINC (mg)
Chocolate wafers (1 wafer)	1	0	2	3	8	0.07
Coconut macaroons, prepared from recipe (1 cookie)	0	0	2	5	10	0.17
Fig (1 cookie)	7	0	10	4	10	0.06
Fortune (1 cookie)	1	0	1	1	3	0.01
Fudge, cake-type (1 cookie)	0	0	7	7	17	0.17
Gingersnaps (1 cookie)	0	0	5	3	6	0.04
Graham crackers, plain or honey, includes cinnamon (2½″ square)	0	0	2	2	7	0.06
Ladyfingers, 1 anisette sponge (4″)	72	1	6	2	23	0.15
Ladyfingers, with lemon juice and rind (1 ladyfinger)	61	0	5	1	19	0.13
Marshmallow, chocolate-coated, includes marshmallow pie (1 pie)	1	1	18	14	38	0.25
Molasses (1 cookie)	0	0	15	10	19	0.09
Oatmeal						
Commercially prepared, fat-free (1 cookie)	0	0	11	10	30	0.18
Commercially prepared, soft-type (1 cookie)	5	0	14	5	31	0.07
Prepared from recipe, with raisins (1 cookie)	96	0	15	6	24	0.13
Peanut butter, prepared from recipe (1 cookie)	120	0	8	8	23	0.16

	VIT A (IU)	VIT C (mg)	CAL (mg)	MAG (mg)	PHOS (mg)	ZINC (mg)
Peanut butter, refrigerated dough (1 cookie)	6	0	13	5	32	0.09
Raisin, soft-type (1 cookie)	6	0	7	3	12	0.05
Shortbread, commercially prepared plain (1 med. cookie)	3	0	3	1	9	0.04
Shortbread, prepared from recipe, made with butter (1 med. cookie)	136	0	2	1	8	0.05
Sugar, prepared from recipe, made with butter, 1 cookie (3″ dia.)	125	0	10	2	13	0.06
Sugar, refrigerated dough, baked (1 cookie)	4	0	11	1	22	0.03
Tea biscuits (2 oz.)	0	0	25	10	65	0.37
Vanilla sandwich, cream filling (1 med. cookie)	0	0	3	1	8	0.04
Vanilla wafers, lower fat (1 med. cookie)	2	0	2	1	4	0.01
Vanilla wafers, higher fat (1 med. cookie)	0	0	2	1	4	0.02

Custards

	VIT A (IU)	VIT C (mg)	CAL (mg)	MAG (mg)	PHOS (mg)	ZINC (mg)
Caramel, flan, dry mix, prepared with 2% milk (½ cup)	249	1	153	17	116	0.48
Caramel, flan, dry mix, prepared with whole milk (½ cup)	153	1	150	16	114	0.47

	VIT A (IU)	VIT C (mg)	CAL (mg)	MAG (mg)	PHOS (mg)	ZINC (mg)
Caramel, flan, prepared from recipe (½ cup)	314	1	132	17	145	0.72
Egg custard						
Dry mix, prepared with 2% milk (½ cup)	295	1	197	27	176	0.71
Dry mix, prepared with whole milk (½ cup)	200	1	194	25	174	0.69
Dry mix, prepared from recipe, 1 piece (⅛ of 9″ dia.)	281	1	107	17	125	0.62

Doughnuts

	VIT A (IU)	VIT C (mg)	CAL (mg)	MAG (mg)	PHOS (mg)	ZINC (mg)
Cake-type						
Chocolate, sugared, glazed, 1 med. (approx. 3″ dia.)	37	0	90	14	68	0.24
Plain, unsugared, old-fashioned, 1 med. (3¼″ dia.)	27	0	21	9	126	0.26
Wheat, sugared or glazed, 1 med. (approx. 3″ dia.)	29	0	22	10	47	0.31
French crullers, glazed (3″ dia.)	7	0	11	5	50	0.12
Yeast-leavened, cream filling 1 med. (3½″ × 2½″ oval)	25	0	21	17	65	0.68
Yeast-leavened, glazed, enriched, includes honey buns (1 bun)	27	0	34	17	73	0.6
Yeast-leavened, with jelly filling, 1 med. (3½″ × 2½″ oval)	26	1	21	17	72	0.64

Frostings	VIT A (IU)	VIT C (mg)	CAL (mg)	MAG (mg)	PHOS (mg)	ZINC (mg)
Chocolate, creamy, prepared from recipe, with margarine (1/12 package)	219	0	9	13	24	0.2
Cream cheese–flavor, ready to eat (1/12 package)	146	0	1	1	1	0
Sour cream–flavor, ready-to-eat (1/12 package)	152	0	1	1	2	0
Vanilla, creamy, ready-to-eat (1/12 package)	284	0	1	0	15	0

Frozen Desserts

	VIT A (IU)	VIT C (mg)	CAL (mg)	MAG (mg)	PHOS (mg)	ZINC (mg)
Fruit and juice bars, 1 bar (3 fl. oz.)	27	9	5	4	6	0.05
Gelatins, dry mix, reduced-calorie, with aspartame (1/2 cup)	0	12	0	0	0	0
Ice cream, chocolate (1/2 cup)	275	1	72	19	71	0.38
Ice cream, chocolate (1 cup)	550	2	144	38	142	0.76
Ice cream, French vanilla, soft-serve (1/2 cup)	464	1	113	10	100	0.45
Ice cream, French vanilla, soft-serve (1 cup)	928	2	226	20	200	0.9
Ice cream, strawberry (1/2 cup)	211	5	79	9	66	0.22
Ice cream, strawberry (1 cup)	422	10	158	18	132	0.44
Ice cream, vanilla (1/2 cup)	270	0	85	9	69	0.46

	VIT A (IU)	VIT C (mg)	CAL (mg)	MAG (mg)	PHOS (mg)	ZINC (mg)
Ice cream, vanilla (1 cup)	540	0	170	18	138	0.92
Ice cream, vanilla, rich (½ cup)	476	1	87	8	70	0.3
Ice cream, vanilla, rich (1 cup)	259	2	174	16	140	0.6
Ice milk, vanilla (½ cup)	109	1	92	10	72	0.29
Ice milk, vanilla (1 cup)	218	2	184	20	144	0.58
Ice milk, vanilla, soft-serve (½ cup)	91	1	138	12	107	0.47
Ice milk, vanilla, soft-serve (1 cup)	182	2	276	24	214	0.94
Italian ice (½ cup)	194	1	1	0	0	0.04
Italian ice (1 cup)	388	2	2	0	0	0.08
Yogurt, chocolate, soft-serve (½ cup)	115	0	106	19	100	0.35
Yogurt, chocolate, soft-serve (1 cup)	230	0	206	38	200	0.7
Yogurt, vanilla, soft-serve (½ cup)	153	1	103	10	93	0.3
Yogurt, vanilla, soft-serve (1 cup)	306	2	206	20	186	0.6

Pastries

	VIT A (IU)	VIT C (mg)	CAL (mg)	MAG (mg)	PHOS (mg)	ZINC (mg)
Ladyfingers (1 ladyfinger)	61	0	5	1	19	0.13
Cream puffs, prepared from recipe, shell, with custard (1 cream puff)	969	0	86	16	142	0.78
Danish, fruit, enriched (1 pastry, 4¼″ dia.)	37	3	33	11	63	0.38
Danish, raspberry, unenriched (1 pastry, 4¼″ dia.)	142	3	33	11	63	0.38

	VIT A (IU)	VIT C (mg)	CAL (mg)	MAG (mg)	PHOS (mg)	ZINC (mg)
Eclair, prepared from recipe, with custard (1 eclair, 5″ × 2″)	671	0	59	11	98	0.54

Pie Crust

	VIT A (IU)	VIT C (mg)	CAL (mg)	MAG (mg)	PHOS (mg)	ZINC (mg)
Cookie-type, prepared from recipe, chocolate wafer, chilled (⅛ of 9″ dia.)	235	0	8	11	29	0.23
Cookie-type, prepared from recipe, graham cracker (⅛ of 9″ dia.)	231	0	6	5	19	0.14
Standard-type, dry mix, prepared, baked (⅛ of 9″ dia.)	0	0	12	3	17	0.8
Standard-type, prepared from recipe (⅛ of 9″ dia.)	0	0	2	3	15	0.1

Pie Fillings

	VIT A (IU)	VIT C (mg)	CAL (mg)	MAG (mg)	PHOS (mg)	ZINC (mg)
Apple, canned (⅛ can)	10	1	3	2	5	0.03
Cherry, canned (⅛ can)	152	3	8	5	11	0.04

Pies

	VIT A (IU)	VIT C (mg)	CAL (mg)	MAG (mg)	PHOS (mg)	ZINC (mg)
Apple, commercially prepared, enriched flour (1 piece, ⅛ of 9″ dia.)	155	4	14	9	30	0.2
Apple, prepared from recipe (1 piece, ⅛ of 9″)	90	3	11	11	43	0.29
Banana cream, prepared from mix no-bake type (1 piece, ⅙ of 8″ dia.)	502	1	90	15	205	0.41

	VIT A (IU)	VIT C (mg)	CAL (mg)	MAG (mg)	PHOS (mg)	ZINC (mg)
Banana cream, prepared from recipe (1 piece, 1/8 of 9″ dia.)	376	2	108	23	133	0.69
Blueberry, prepared from recipe (1 piece, 1/8 of 9″ dia.)	62	1	10	12	44	0.29
Butterscotch, pudding-type, prepared from recipe (1 piece, 1/8 of 9″ dia.)	382	1	128	22	135	0.69
Cherry, prepared from recipe, (1 piece 1/8 of 9″)	736	2	18	16	54	0.36
Chocolate cream, prepared from recipe (1 piece, 1/8 of 9″ dia.)	375	1	115	37	156	0.91
Coconut cream, prepared from mix, no-bake type (1 piece, 1/8 of 9″ dia.)	381	1	68	16	159	0.36
Coconut cream, prepared from recipe (1 piece, 1/8 of 9″ dia.)	380	1	113	21	140	0.81
Fried, cherry, 1 fried pie (5″ × 3¾″)	220	2	28	13	55	0.29
Lemon meringue, commercially prepared (1 piece, 1/6 of 8″ dia.)	198	4	63	17	119	0.55
Lemon meringue, prepared from recipe (1 piece, 1/8 of 9″ dia.)	203	4	15	8	53	0.36
Mince, prepared from recipe, (1 piece 1/8 of 9″)	36	10	36	23	69	0.36

	VIT A (IU)	VIT C (mg)	CAL (mg)	MAG (mg)	PHOS (mg)	ZINC (mg)
Peach (1 piece, ⅙ of 8″ dia.)	123	1	9	7	29	0.11
Pecan, prepared from recipe, (1 piece ⅛ of 9″)	410	0	39	32	115	1.24
Pumpkin, prepared from recipe, (1 piece, ⅛ of 9″ dia.)	11,833	3	146	30	152	0.71
Vanilla cream, prepared from recipe (1 piece, ⅛ of 9″ dia.)	386	1	113	16	131	0.67

Puddings

	VIT A (IU)	VIT C (mg)	CAL (mg)	MAG (mg)	PHOS (mg)	ZINC (mg)
Banana, dry mix, instant, prepared with 2% milk (½ cup)	250	2	150	18	318	0.49
Banana, dry mix, instant, prepared with whole milk (½ cup)	154	1	147	18	315	0.47
Banana, dry mix, regular, prepared with 2% milk (½ cup)	252	1	154	18	118	0.5
Bread, prepared from recipe (½ cup)	304	1	144	24	137	0.66
Chocolate, dry mix, instant, prepared, with 2% milk (½ cup)	253	1	153	27	353	0.65
Chocolate, dry mix, instant, prepared with whole milk (½ cup)	157	1	150	27	351	0.62
Chocolate, dry mix, regular, prepared with 2% milk (½ cup)	253	1	161	30	138	0.65

	VIT A (IU)	VIT C (mg)	CAL (mg)	MAG (mg)	PHOS (mg)	ZINC (mg)
Chocolate, dry mix, regular, prepared with whole milk (½ cup)	156	1	158	21	132	0.64
Chocolate, prepared from recipe with 2% milk (½ cup)	291	1	155	39	149	0.79
Chocolate, prepared from recipe with whole milk (½ cup)	193	1	153	38	148	0.77
Lemon, dry mix, instant, with 2% milk (½ cup)	250	1	149	16	304	0.49
Lemon, dry mix, instant, with whole milk (½ cup)	154	1	146	16	301	0.47
Rice, dry mix, prepared with 2% milk (½ cup)	249	1	151	19	127	0.56
Rice, dry mix, prepared with whole milk (½ cup)	154	1	148	19	124	0.55
Rice, prepared from recipe (½ cup)	154	1	155	24	143	0.68
Tapioca, dry mix, prepared with 2% milk (½ cup)	251	1	150	17	117	0.49
Tapioca, dry mix, prepared with whole milk (½ cup)	154	1	147	17	116	0.48
Tapioca, prepared from recipe (½ cup)	315	1	158	20	160	0.75
Tapioca, ready-to-eat (½ cup)	0	1	95	9	89	0.31
Vanilla						
Dry mix, instant, prepared with 2% milk (½ cup)	241	1	146	17	183	0.47

	VIT A (IU)	VIT C (mg)	CAL (mg)	MAG (mg)	PHOS (mg)	ZINC (mg)
Dry mix, regular, prepared with 2% milk (½ cup)	252	1	153	18	118	0.5
Dry mix, regular, prepared with whole milk (½ cup)	154	1	150	18	115	0.49
Ready-to-eat (½ cup)	24	0	99	9	77	0.28

Toppings

Butterscotch (2 tbsp.)	37	0	22	3	19	0.08
Caramel (2 tbsp.)	37	0	22	3	19	0.08
Chocolate syrup, prepared with milk (1 cup)	1126	2	292	32	229	0.92
Cream topping, whipped, pressurized (1 cup)	548	0	61	7	54	0.22
Dessert topping, powdered, 1.5 oz. (1 cup prepared)	289	1	72	8	67	0.22
Marshmallow cream (1 oz.)	0	0	1	1	2	0.01
Nuts in syrup (2 tbsp.)	17	1	16	26	46	0.43
Pineapple (2 tbsp.)	9	25	9	1	3	0.2
Rainbow Morsel Dessert Topping, Nestlé (1 packet)	1	0	4	11	13	0.15
Strawberry (2 tbsp.)	8	11	10	2	6	0.21

EGGS

Raw, whole, fresh or frozen (1 large egg)	318	0	25	5	89	0.55
White, fresh or frozen (from 1 large egg)	0	0	2	4	4	0

	VIT A (IU)	VIT C (mg)	CAL (mg)	MAG (mg)	PHOS (mg)	ZINC (mg)
Yolk, fresh or frozen (from 1 large egg)	323	0	23	1	81	0.52
Egg Beaters (¼ cup)	300	0	20	*	*	*
Morningstar Farms Better'n Eggs (¼ cup)	640	0	7	0	29	0.51
Vegetarian, frozen (2 oz.)	311	0	2	4	4	0
Second Nature Eggs, yellow carton (¼ cup)	600	0	20	*	*	*
Second Nature Eggs, green carton (¼ cup)	500	0	40	*	*	*

FAST FOODS

Beverages

	VIT A (IU)	VIT C (mg)	CAL (mg)	MAG (mg)	PHOS (mg)	ZINC (mg)
Chocolate, hot (6 oz.)	4	1	96	25	89	0.46
Float (10 oz.)	*	*	200	*	*	*
Juice, orange (6 oz.)	146	73	17	19	30	0.09
Juice, tomato (6 oz.)	1012	33	16	20	34	0.26
Malt (10 oz.)	270	4	400	*	*	*
Shakes						
Chocolate (10 oz.)	263	1	319	47	288	1.15
Strawberry (10 oz.)	340	2	320	36	283	1
Vanilla (10 oz.)	368	2	344	35	289	1.01

Breakfast

	VIT A (IU)	VIT C (mg)	CAL (mg)	MAG (mg)	PHOS (mg)	ZINC (mg)
Biscuits						
Egg (1 biscuit)	649	0	154	20	185	1.1
Egg and bacon (1 biscuit)	191	3	189	24	239	1.64
Egg, cheese, and bacon (1 biscuit)	648	2	164	20	459	1.54
Ham (1 biscuit)	133	0	161	23	554	1.65
Sausage (1 biscuit)	56	0	128	20	446	1.55

	VIT A (IU)	VIT C (mg)	CAL (mg)	MAG (mg)	PHOS (mg)	ZINC (mg)
Burrito (1 burrito)	1000	0	350	*	*	*
Croissant						
Egg and cheese (1 croissant)	1001	0	244	22	348	1.75
Egg, cheese, and bacon (1 croissant)	472	2	151	23	276	1.9
Egg, cheese, and sausage (1 croissant)	422	0	144	25	290	2.15
Danish						
Cheese (1 pastry)	155	3	70	16	80	0.63
Fruit (1 pastry)	86	2	22	14	69	0.48
Egg, scrambled (2 eggs)	836	3	54	13	228	1.56
English muffin						
Butter (1 muffin)	136	1	103	13	85	0.42
Egg, cheese, and Canadian bacon (1 muffin)	594	1	207	34	320	1.81
Egg, cheese, and sausage (1 muffin)	380	1	168	24	186	1.68
French toast sticks (5 pieces)	45	0	78	27	123	0.93
Pancakes with butter and syrup (2 cakes)	281	4	128	49	476	1.02

Desserts

	VIT A (IU)	VIT C (mg)	CAL (mg)	MAG (mg)	PHOS (mg)	ZINC (mg)
Apple pie, baked (1 slice)	500	1	20	6	*	*
Banana split (1 serving)	0	18	300	*	*	*
Brownie (2″ square)	11	3	25	16	88	0.55
Cookie						
Animal crackers (1 box)	27	1	11	11	64	0.3

	VIT A (IU)	VIT C (mg)	CAL (mg)	MAG (mg)	PHOS (mg)	ZINC (mg)
Chocolate chip (1 box)	52	1	20	17	52	0.34
Fried pie, fruit, apple, cherry, or lemon (1 fried pie)	149	1	13	8	37	0.17
Ice cream cone, regular (1 cone)	135	3	150	21	*	*
Ice milk, vanilla, soft-serve, with cone (1 cone)	211	1	154	16	139	0.57
Sundae						
Caramel (1 sundae)	264	3	189	28	217	0.82
Hot fudge (1 sundae)	221	2	207	33	228	0.95
Strawberry (1 sundae)	222	2	161	25	155	0.66

Entrées

	VIT A (IU)	VIT C (mg)	CAL (mg)	MAG (mg)	PHOS (mg)	ZINC (mg)
Chicken						
Breaded and fried, boneless pieces, plain (6 pieces)	102	0	16	20	204	1.06
Breaded and fried, boneless pieces with barbecue sauce (6 pieces)	342	1	21	25	215	1.12
Breaded and fried, light meat breast or wing (2 pieces)	192	0	60	38	306	1.55
Chili con carne (1 cup)	1662	2	68	46	197	3.57
Clams, breaded and fried (¾ cup)	122	0	21	31	238	1.63
Crab, soft-shell, fried (1 crab)	15	1	55	25	131	1.06
Oysters, battered or breaded and fried (6 pieces)	363	4	28	24	196	15.6

	VIT A (IU)	VIT C (mg)	CAL (mg)	MAG (mg)	PHOS (mg)	ZINC (mg)
Scallops, breaded and fried (6 pieces)	138	0	19	32	292	1.08
Shrimp, breaded and fried (6–8 pieces)	120	0	84	39	344	1.21
Burrito						
Beans and cheese (1 piece)	1250	2	214	80	180	1.64
Beans and meat (2 pieces)	635	2	106	84	141	3.84
Beans, cheese, and chili peppers (2 pieces)	1596	7	289	97	286	6.08
Beans, cheese, and beans (2 pieces)	780	5	130	51	140	2.36
Chimichanga, with beef, cheese, and red chili peppers (1 chimichanga)	702	2	218	41	148	4.63
Enchilada, with cheese (1 enchilada)	1161	1	324	51	134	2.51
Enchirito, with cheese, beef, and cheese (1 enchilada or enchirito)	1015	5	218	71	224	1.74
Taco (1 large)	1315	3	339	108	313	6.05
Tostada, with beans and cheese (1 piece)	622	1	210	59	117	1.9

Pizza

	VIT A (IU)	VIT C (mg)	CAL (mg)	MAG (mg)	PHOS (mg)	ZINC (mg)
Beef (1 slice)	450	*	115	*	*	*
Cheese (1 slice)	382	1	117	16	113	0.81
Cheese, meat, and vegetables (1 slice)	524	2	101	18	131	1.12
Italian sausage (1 slice)	450	*	110	*	*	*
Pepperoni (1 slice)	282	2	65	9	75	0.52
Veggie (1 slice)	500	0	110	*	*	*

Salads	VIT A (IU)	VIT C (mg)	CAL (mg)	MAG (mg)	PHOS (mg)	ZINC (mg)
Coleslaw (¾ cup)	338	8	34	9	36	0.2
Taco (1½ cups)	588	4	192	52	143	2.69
Taco, with chili con carne (1½ cups)	1574	3	245	52	154	3.29
Vegetable salad						
Tossed, without dressing (1½ cups)	2352	48	27	23	81	0.44
Tossed, without dressing, with cheese and egg (1½ cups)	822	10	100	24	132	1
Tossed, without dressing, with chicken (1½ cups)	935	17	37	33	170	0.89
Tossed, without dressing, with pasta and seafood (1½ cups)	6247	38	71	50	204	1.67
Tossed, without dressing, with shrimp (1½ cups)	791	9	59	38	161	1.27
Tossed, without dressing, with turkey, ham, and cheese (1½ cups)	1053	16	235	49	401	3.13
Sandwiches						
Cheeseburger						
Patty, double, large, with condiments (1 sandwich)	462	2	111	20	176	2.09
Patty, double, large, with condiments and vegetables (1 sandwich)	348	1	240	52	395	6.68

	VIT A (IU)	VIT C (mg)	CAL (mg)	MAG (mg)	PHOS (mg)	ZINC (mg)
Patty, single, regular, with condiments and vegetables (1 sandwich)	431	2	182	26	216	2.62
Chicken, broiled (1 sandwich)	150	6	75	30	*	*
Chicken fillet sandwich, plain (1 sandwich)	100	9	60	35	233	1.88
Chicken fillet, with cheese (1 sandwich)	620	3	258	43	406	2.9
Egg and cheese (1 sandwich)	669	2	225	22	302	1.65
Fish, with tartar sauce (1 sandwich)	109	3	84	33	212	1
Fish, with tartar sauce and cheese (1 sandwich)	432	3	185	37	311	1.17
Ham and cheese (1 sandwich)	320	3	130	16	152	1.37
Hot dog, plain (1 sandwich)	0	0	24	13	97	1.98
Hot dog, with corn flour coating, corn dog (1 sandwich)	207	0	102	18	166	1.31
Roast beef, plain (1 sandwich)	210	2	54	31	239	3.39
Submarine						
Cold cuts (1 sandwich)	424	12	189	68	287	2.58
Roast beef (1 sandwich)	413	6	41	67	192	4.39
Tuna salad (1 sandwich)	187	4	74	79	335	1.87

Side dishes

	VIT A (IU)	VIT C (mg)	CAL (mg)	MAG (mg)	PHOS (mg)	ZINC (mg)
Corn, on the cob with butter (1 ear)	391	7	4	41	108	0.91

	VIT A (IU)	VIT C (mg)	CAL (mg)	MAG (mg)	PHOS (mg)	ZINC (mg)
Hush puppies (5 pieces)	94	0	69	16	190	0.43
Nachos						
Cheese (6–8 nachos)	559	1	272	55	276	1.79
Cheese and jalapeño peppers (6–8 nachos)	4062	1	620	108	394	2.9
Cheese, beans, ground beef, and peppers (6–8 nachos)	3401	5	385	97	388	3.65
Cinnamon and sugar (6–8 nachos)	108	8	85	20	33	0.59
Onion rings, breaded and fried (8–9 rings)	8	1	73	16	86	0.35
Potato						
Baked and topped with cheese, sauce (1 piece)	835	26	311	65	320	1.89
Baked and topped with cheese, sauce, and bacon (1 piece)	628	29	308	69	347	2.15
Baked and topped with cheese, sauce, and broccoli (1 piece)	1695	49	336	78	346	2.03
Baked and topped with cheese, sauce, and chili (1 piece)	766	32	411	111	498	3.79
Baked and topped with sour cream and chives (1 piece)	1347	34	106	70	184	0.91
French fried in vegetable oil (1 large potato)	33	6	18	38	153	0.6
Mashed (⅓ cup)	33	0	17	14	44	0.26

FATS	VIT A (IU)	VIT C (mg)	CAL (mg)	MAG (mg)	PHOS (mg)	ZINC (mg)
Butter						
Blend, corn oil and butter (1 tbsp.)	507	0	4	0	3	0
Regular (1 tbsp.)	434	0	3	0	3	0.01
Whipped (1 tbsp.)	288	0	2	0	2	0.01
Margarine/Spreads						
Hard, soybean, regular, hydrogenated (1 tsp.)	168	0	1	0	1	0
Imitation, soybean, hydrogenated (1 tsp.)	171	0	1	0	1	0
Liquid, soybean and cottonseed, hydrogenated and regular (1 tsp.)	168	0	3	0	2	0
Soft, corn, hydrogenated and regular (1 tsp.)	168	0	1	0	1	0
Soft, soybean, hydrogenated and regular (1 tsp.)	168	0	1	0	1	0
Soft spread, Smart Balance, GFA Brands (1 tbsp.)	500	*	*	*	*	*
Soybean, soft, hydrogenated and regular (1 tsp.)	168	0	1	0	1	0
Spread, tub, soybean and cottonseed oil, hydrogenated (1 tsp.)	171	0	1	0	1	0

Mayonnaise	VIT A (IU)	VIT C (mg)	CAL (mg)	MAG (mg)	PHOS (mg)	ZINC (mg)
Imitation, milk cream (1 tbsp.)	2	0	11	1	9	0.04
Imitation, soybean (1 tbsp.)	0	0	0	0	0	0.02
Imitation, soybean, without cholesterol (1 tbsp.)	0	0	0	0	0	0.02
Regular (1 tbsp.)	32	0	2	0	4	0.03
Soybean oil (1 tbsp.)	39	0	3	0	4	0.02
Oil						
Canola (1 tbsp.)	0	0	0	0	0	0
Corn, salad or cooking (1 tbsp.)	0	0	0	0	0	0
Cottonseed, salad or cooking (1 tbsp.)	0	0	0	0	0	0
Olive, salad or cooking (1 tbsp.)	0	0	0	0	0	0.01
Peanut, salad or cooking (1 tbsp.)	0	0	0	0	0	0
Safflower, salad or cooking (1 tbsp.)	0	0	0	0	0	0
Sesame, salad or cooking (1 tbsp.)	0	0	0	0	0	0
Soybean, salad or cooking, hydrogenated (1 tbsp.)	0	0	0	0	0	0
Sunflower (1 tbsp.)	0	0	0	0	0	0
Tomatoseed (1 tbsp.)	0	0	0	0	0	0
Wheat germ (1 tbsp.)	0	0	0	0	0	0

FRUIT

	VIT A (IU)	VIT C (mg)	CAL (mg)	MAG (mg)	PHOS (mg)	ZINC (mg)
Acerola, West Indian cherry, raw (1 cup)	752	1655	12	18	11	0.09

	VIT A (IU)	VIT C (mg)	CAL (mg)	MAG (mg)	PHOS (mg)	ZINC (mg)
Apples						
Dried, uncooked (1 ring)	0	0	1	1	2	0.01
Frozen, unsweetened (1 cup)	59	0	7	5	14	0.09
Raw, with skin (1 medium)	73	8	10	7	10	0.06
Apricots						
Dried, stewed, without sugar (½ cup)	2954	2	20	22	52	0.33
Dried, stewed, without sugar (1 cup)	5908	4	40	43	103	0.65
Frozen, sweeten (1 cup)	4066	22	24	22	46	0.24
Raw (1 apricot)	914	4	5	3	7	0.09
Avocados, raw (1 cup)	894	12	16	57	60	0.61
Bananas, raw (½ medium)	48	6	4	17	12	0.099
Bananas, raw (1 medium)	96	11	7	34	24	0.19
Blackberries						
Frozen, unsweetened (½ cup)	86	2.5	22	17	23	0.29
Frozen, unsweetened (1 cup)	172	5	44	33	45	0.38
Raw (½ cup)	129	15	23	15	15	0.19
Raw (1 cup)	238	30	46	29	30	0.39
Blueberries						
Frozen, sweetened (1 cup)	101	2	14	5	16	0.14
Frozen, unsweetened (½ cup)	63	2	6	4	8.5	0.06
Frozen, unsweetened (1 cup)	126	4	12	8	17	0.11
Raw (½ cup)	73	9	5	4	8	0.08

	VIT A (IU)	VIT C (mg)	CAL (mg)	MAG (mg)	PHOS (mg)	ZINC (mg)
Raw (1 cup)	145	19	9	7	15	0.16
Breadfruit, raw (¼ small fruit)	38	28	16	24	29	0.12
Cantaloupe, raw (1 cup cubes)	5158	68	18	18	27	0.26
Casaba, raw (1 cup cubes)	51	27	9	14	12	0.27
Cherimoya, raw, without skin and seeds (1 fruit)	55	49	126	218	*	*
Cherries						
Sour, red, raw without pits (1 cup)	1989	16	25	14	23	0.16
Sweet, raw, without pits (1 cup)	310	10	22	16	28	0.09
Sweet, frozen, thawed (1 cup)	490	3	31	26	41	0.1
Coconut meat, raw (1 cup shredded)	0	3	11	26	90	0.88
Crabapples, raw (1 cup slices)	44	9	20	8	17	*
Currants, European black, raw (1 cup)	258	203	62	27	66	0.3
Currants, red and white, raw (1 cup)	134	46	37	15	49	0.26
Dates, domestic, natural and dry (1 cup, pitted)	89	0	57	62	71	0.52
Figs, dried, stewed (1 cup)	412	11	158	65	75	0.54
Figs, raw (1 medium)	71	1	18	9	7	0.08

	VIT A (IU)	VIT C (mg)	CAL (mg)	MAG (mg)	PHOS (mg)	ZINC (mg)
Fruit, mixed, peach, cherry (sweet and sour), raspberry, grape, and boysenberry, frozen, sweetened (1 cup thawed)	805	188	18	15	30	0.13
Gooseberries, raw (1 cup)	435	42	38	15	41	0.18
Grapefruit, raw, pink, red, and white, all areas (½ large)	206	57	20	13	13	0.12
Grapes, American type, slip skin, raw (1 cup)	92	4	13	5	9	0.04
Honeydew, raw (1 cup, diced)	68	42	10	12	17	0.12
Jackfruit, raw (100 g)	297	6.7	34	37	36	0.42
Kiwi fruit, Chinese gooseberries, raw (1 large fruit without skin)	160	90	24	27	36	0.16
Mangos, raw (1 cup, sliced)	6425	46	17	15	18	0.07
Mulberries, raw (1 cup)	35	51	55	25	53	0.17
Nectarines, raw (1 cup, sliced)	1016	7	7	11	22	0.12
Oranges, raw (1 fruit)	269	70	52	13	18	0.09
Papayas, raw (1 medium)	863	188	73	30	15	0.21
Passion fruit, purple, raw (1 fruit, sliced)	126	5	2	5	12	0.02
Peaches						
Dried, stewed, without sugar (1 cup)	508	10	23	34	98	0.46
Raw (1 medium)	524	7	5	7	12	0.14

	VIT A (IU)	VIT C (mg)	CAL (mg)	MAG (mg)	PHOS (mg)	ZINC (mg)
Frozen, sliced, sweetened (1 cup, thawed)	710	236	8	13	28	0.13
Pears, dried, stewed, without added sugar (1 cup, halves)	107	10	41	41	71	0.49
Pears, raw (1 medium pear)	33	7	18	10	18	0.2
Plantains, cooked (1 cup, sliced)	1400	17	3	49	43	0.2
Plantains, raw (1 cup, sliced)	1668	27	4	55	50	0.2
Plums, raw (1 fruit)	213	6	3	5	7	0.07
Pomegranates, raw (1 fruit)	0	9	5	5	12	0.19
Prunes, dehydrated, uncooked (1 cup)	2326	0	95	85	148	0.99
Prunes, dried, stewed, without sugar (1 cup, pitted)	759	7	57	50	87	0.6
Raisins, golden seedless (1 cup)	64	5	77	51	167	0.46
Raisins, seedless (1 cup, not packed)	12	5	71	48	141	0.39
Raspberries, frozen, red, sweetened (1 cup, unthawed)	150	41	38	33	43	0.45
Raspberries, raw (1 cup)	160	31	27	22	15	0.57
Rhubarb, frozen, cooked, with sugar (1 cup)	166	8	348	29	19	0.19
Rhubarb, raw (1 cup, diced)	122	10	105	15	17	0.12
Strawberries, frozen, sweetened, whole (1 cup, thawed)	69	101	28	15	31	0.13

	VIT A (IU)	VIT C (mg)	CAL (mg)	MAG (mg)	PHOS (mg)	ZINC (mg)
Strawberries, frozen, unsweetened (1 cup, thawed)	100	91	35	24	29	0.29
Strawberries, raw (1 cup, whole)	39	82	20	14	27	0.19
Tamarindo, tart date-apricot flavored fruit (3 oz.)	0	4	60	*	*	*
Tangerines, raw (1 medium)	773	26	12	10	8	0.2
Watermelon, raw (1 cup, diced)	556	15	12	17	14	0.11

Canned Fruit

	VIT A (IU)	VIT C (mg)	CAL (mg)	MAG (mg)	PHOS (mg)	ZINC (mg)
Apples, sweetened, sliced, drained (1 cup)	104	1	8	4	10	0.06
Applesauce, sweetened (1 cup)	28	4	10	8	18	0.1
Apricots, juice pack, with skin (1 cup, halves)	4126	12	29	24	49	0.27
Apricots, water pack, with skin (1 cup)	3142	8	19	17	32	0.27
Blackberries, heavy syrup (1 cup)	561	7	54	44	35	0.46
Blueberries, heavy syrup (1 cup)	164	3	13	10	26	0.18
Cherries, sour, red, light syrup pack (1 cup)	1830	5	25	15	25	0.18
Cherries, sour, red, water pack, solids and liquids (1 cup)	1840	5	27	15	24	0.17
Cherries, sweet, water pack (1 cup)	397	5	27	22	37	0.2

	VIT A (IU)	VIT C (mg)	CAL (mg)	MAG (mg)	PHOS (mg)	ZINC (mg)
Figs, light syrup pack (1 cup)	93	3	68	25	25	0.28
Fruit cocktail, peach, pineapple, pear, grape, and cherry, juice packed (1 cup)	723	6	19	17	33	0.21
Fruit salad, peach, pear, apricot, pineapple, and cherry, juice pack (1 cup)	1494	8	27	20	35	0.35
Gooseberries, light syrup pack (1 cup)	348	25	40	15	18	0.28
Grapefruit, sections, juice pack (1 cup)	0	84	37	27	30	0.2
Orange-grapefruit juice, unsweetened (1 cup)	294	72	20	25	35	0.17
Papaya nectar (1 cup)	278	8	25	8	0	0.37
Peaches, juice pack (1 cup)	945	9	15	17	42	0.27
Pears, juice pack (1 cup)	5	1	7	5	9	0.07
Pineapple, juice pack (1 cup)	95	24	35	35	15	0.25
Plums, purple, juice pack (1 cup, pitted)	2543	7	25	20	38	0.28
Raspberries, red, heavy syrup (1 cup)	85	22	28	31	23	0.41
Strawberries, heavy syrup pack (1 cup)	66	81	33	20	31	0.23
Tangerines (or mandarin oranges), juice pack (1 cup)	2122	85	27	27	25	1.27

FRUIT JUICES

	VIT A (IU)	VIT C (mg)	CAL (mg)	MAG (mg)	PHOS (mg)	ZINC (mg)
Apple cider, canned (1 cup)	*	6000	*	*	*	*

	VIT A (IU)	VIT C (mg)	CAL (mg)	MAG (mg)	PHOS (mg)	ZINC (mg)
Apple juice						
Canned, unsweetened, with added ascorbic acid (1 cup)	3	103	17	7	17	0.07
Canned, unsweetened, canned (1 cup)	3	2	17	7	17	0.07
Frozen concentrate (1 cup)	0	60	14	12	17	0.1
Apricot nectar, canned (1 cup)	3304	1	17	13	23	0.23
Carrot juice, canned (1 cup)	60,772	20	57	33	99	0.43
Carrot, Apple, and Tropical Fruit Blend, V-8, 25% juice (1 cup)	5000	60	*	*	*	*
Citrus fruit juice drink, frozen concentrate, prepared (1 cup)	104	67	22	15	25	0.12
Clam and tomato juice, canned (1 can, 5.5 oz.)	357	7	20	37	130	1.79
Cranberry-apple juice drink, bottled (1 cup)	7	78	17	5	7	0.1
Cranberry-apricot juice drink, bottled (1 cup)	1134	0	22	7	12	0.1
Cranberry-grape juice drink, bottled (1 cup)	12	78	20	7	10	0.1
Cranberry juice cocktail, bottled (1 cup)	10	90	8	5	5	0.18
Cranberry juice cocktail, bottled, low calorie, with calcium (1 cup)	10	76	21	5	2	0.05

	VIT A (IU)	VIT C (mg)	CAL (mg)	MAG (mg)	PHOS (mg)	ZINC (mg)
Cranberry juice cocktail, frozen, concentrate, prepared (1 cup)	25	25	13	5	3	0.1
Grape juice, canned or bottled, unsweetened, without added vitamin C (1 cup)	20	0	23	25	28	0.13
Grape juice, frozen concentrate, sweetened (1 cup)	20	60	10	10	10	0.1
Grape juice drink, canned (1 cup)	5	40	8	10	10	0.08
Grapefruit juice, canned, sweetened (1 cup)	0	67	20	25	28	0.15
Grapefruit juice, frozen concentrate, unsweetened, undiluted (1 can, 6 oz.)	64	248	56	79	101	0.37
Grapefruit juice, pink, raw (1 cup)	1087	94	22	30	37	0.12
Grapefruit juice, white, raw (1 cup)	25	94	22	30	37	0.12
Lemonade, powder, prepared with water (1 cup)	0	8	71	3	34	0.11
Lemon juice, canned or bottled (1 oz.)	5	8	3	2	3	0.02
Lemon juice, raw (juice of 1 lemon)	9	22	3	3	3	0.02
Lime juice, canned or bottled, unsweetened (1 oz.)	5	2	4	2	3	0.02
Lime juice, raw (1 oz.)	3	9	3	2	2	0.02
Orange-apricot juice drink, canned (1 cup)	1450	50	13	10	20	0.13

	VIT A (IU)	VIT C (mg)	CAL (mg)	MAG (mg)	PHOS (mg)	ZINC (mg)
Orange-grapefruit juice, canned, unsweetened (1 cup)	294	72	20	25	35	0.17
Orange juice						
Canned, unsweetened (1 cup)	435	86	20	26	35	0.17
From concentrate, Season's Best, Tropicana (1 cup)	0	60	300	*	*	*
Frozen concentrate, unsweetened, diluted with water (1 cup)	194	97	22	25	40	0.13
Raw (1 cup)	496	124	27	27	42	0.12
Squeezed, Not From Concentrate Plus Calcium, Florida's Natural Brand, Citrus World (1 cup)	*	108	350	31	41	.01
Squeezed, Not from Concentrate Calcium Enriched, Tropicana (1 cup)	*	108	350	*	*	*
Papaya nectar, canned (1 cup)	278	8	25	8	0	0.38
Passion fruit juice, raw (1 cup)	1771	74	10	42	32	0.12
Passion fruit juice, yellow, raw (1 cup)	5953	45	10	42	62	0.15
Peach nectar, canned, with ascorbic acid (1 cup)	642	67	13	10	15	0.2
Pear nectar, canned, with added ascorbic acid (1 cup)	3	68	13	8	8	0.18

	VIT A (IU)	VIT C (mg)	CAL (mg)	MAG (mg)	PHOS (mg)	ZINC (mg)
Pineapple juice, canned, with added ascorbic acid, unsweetened (1 cup)	13	60	43	33	20	0.28
Pineapple juice, frozen concentrate, unsweetened, diluted with water (1 cup)	25	30	28	23	20	0.28
Pineapple-grapefruit juice drink, canned (1 cup)	88	115	18	15	15	0.15
Pineapple-orange juice drink, canned (1 cup)	1328	56	13	15	10	0.15
Prune juice, canned (1 cup)	8	11	31	36	64	0.54
Tangerine juice, canned, sweetened (1 cup)	1046	55	45	20	35	0.08
Tangerine juice, frozen concentrate sweetened, diluted with water (1 cup)	1381	59	19	19	19	0.07
Tangerine juice, frozen concentrate sweetened, undiluted (6 oz.)	4310	182	58	60	64	0.19
Tangerine juice, raw (1 cup)	1037	77	45	20	35	0.07
Tomato juice, canned, with salt added (1 cup)	1351	45	22	27	46	0.34
Tomato juice, canned, without salt added (1 cup)	1351	45	22	27	46	0.34

	VIT A (IU)	VIT C (mg)	CAL (mg)	MAG (mg)	PHOS (mg)	ZINC (mg)
Vegetable juice cocktail, canned (1 cup)	2831	67	27	27	41	0.48

GRAVIES, SAUCES, AND DIPS

Gravies

Au jus, canned (1 cup)	0	2	10	5	72	2.38
Beef, canned (1 cup)	0	0	14	5	70	2.33
Chicken, canned (1 cup)	878	0	48	5	69	1.9
Mushroom, canned (1 cup)	0	0	17	5	36	1.67
Turkey gravy mix, canned (1 cup)	0	0	10	5	70	2
Turkey Gravy Mix, Nestlé, Trio, dry (1 serving)	0	0	10	5	29	0.01

Sauces

Alfredo, dry, Nestlé, Trio (100 g)	567	0	467	32	415	1.49
Barbecue (1 packet)	81	1	2	2	2	0.02
Béarnaise, dehydrated, dry (1 cup)	1	0	27	5	24	0.12
Cheese						
Cheddar, basic, Nestlé, Chef-Mate ready-to-serve (¼ cup)	39	1	46	4	51	0.34
Jalapeño, Nestlé, Que Bueno (¼ cup)	71	1	54	4	52	0.34
Mix, dry, Nestlé, Trio (2 tbsp.)	21	0	22	4	34	0.13
Sharp cheddar, Nestlé, Chef-Mate ready-to-serve (1 cup)	1210	0	544	25	421	2.6

	VIT A (IU)	VIT C (mg)	CAL (mg)	MAG (mg)	PHOS (mg)	ZINC (mg)
Chili, hot dog sauce, ready-to-serve Nestlé, Chef-Mate (¼ cup)	423	0	20	13	40	0.55
Cranberry sauce, canned, sweetened (1 slice)	11	1	2	2	3	0.03
Creole, ready-to-serve, Nestlé, Chef-Mate (¼ cup)	234	0	35	9	17	0.1
Curry, dehydrated, dry (1 cup)	29	1	50	12	42	0.26
Enchilada, ready-to-serve, Nestlé, Que Bueno (2 tbsp.)	123	2	7	5	11	0.06
Guava, cooked (1 cup)	674	348	17	17	26	0.41
Hollandaise, with butterfat, dehydrated, dry (1 packet)	573	0	97	6	99	0.54
Lemon, ready-to-serve, Nestlé, Chef-Mate (2 tbsp.)	0	3	1	1	1	0.01
Marinara, ready-to-serve (½ cup)	469	10	28	21	40	0.21
Pesto (¼ package)	300	*	20	*	*	*
Plum, ready-to-serve (1 tbsp.)	8	0	2	2	4	0.04
Sour cream, dehydrated, dry (1 tbsp.)	85	0	128	7	42	0.64
Spaghetti sauce, ready-to-serve, Nestlé, Contadine (½ cup)	500	11	31	28	46	0.26
Stir fry sauce, Nestlé, Chef-Mate, all purpose (1 tbsp.)	4	1	2	2	5	0.02

	VIT A (IU)	VIT C (mg)	CAL (mg)	MAG (mg)	PHOS (mg)	ZINC (mg)
Stroganoff, dehydrated, dry (1 cup)	268	0	371	23	152	1.33
Sweet and sour, dehydrated, dry (1 cup)	0	0	41	9	45	0.09
Szechuan, ready-to-serve, Nestlé Chef-Mate (2 tbsp.)	197	1	4	3	12	0.04
Teriyaki, ready-to-serve, Nestlé, Chef-Mate (1 tbsp.)	0	0	1	1	3	0.02
Tomato, canned (1 cup)	2399	32	34	47	78	0.61
White, homemade sauce						
Medium (½ cup)	691	1	148	18	123	0.51
Thick (½ cup)	841	1	139	18	120	0.5
Thin (½ cup)	504	1	158	19	126	0.53
Dips						
Cheese, prepared (1 cup)	1473	2	756	46	557	0.06
Cheese, fondue (1 cup)	890	0	1023	50	658	4.21
Con Queso, Nestlé, Que Bueno (¼ cup)	172	0	118	4	52	0.33
Garden vegetable, prepared (1 tbsp.)	200	2	40	*	*	*
Nacho, Nestlé, Que Bueno (¼ cup)	481	0	181	6	105	0.65
Ranch, fat-free, prepared with fat-free sour cream (1/16 packet)	200	0	60	*	*	*
Ranch, prepared (1/16 packet)	200	0	20	*	*	*
Picante, ready-to-serve, Nestlé, Que Bueno (2 tbsp.)	83	1	13	5	8	0.05

	VIT A (IU)	VIT C (mg)	CAL (mg)	MAG (mg)	PHOS (mg)	ZINC (mg)
Salsa, creamy, fat-free, prepared (2 tbsp.)	*	*	60	*	*	*
Salsa, ready-to-serve (½ cup)	862	26	60	16	30	0.38

MEATS

Beef

	VIT A (IU)	VIT C (mg)	CAL (mg)	MAG (mg)	PHOS (mg)	ZINC (mg)
Brisket, whole, lean and fat, all grades, braised (3 oz.)	0	0	7	15	159	4.34
Chuck, arm pot roast, lean and fat, choice, braised (3 oz.)	0	0	9	16	184	5.7
Chuck, blade roast, lean and fat, choice, braised (3 oz.)	0	0	15	26	223	9.23
Corn beef, cured, canned (100 g)	0	0	12	14	106	3.87
Flank, lean only, choice, braised (3 oz.)	0	0	5	20	227	5.14
Ground, lean, pan-fried, medium (3 oz.)	0	0	6	18	136	4.61
Liver, braised (3 oz.)	30,327	20	6	17	343	5.16
Liver, pan-fried (3 oz.)	30,589	20	9	20	392	4.63
Porterhouse short loin, steak, lean, choice, broiled (3 oz.)	0	0	6	23	179	4.5
Porterhouse steak, short loin, lean and fat, choice, broiled (3 oz.)	0	0	7	19	152	3.7
Rib eye, small end (ribs 10–12), lean and fat, choice, broiled (3 oz.)	3	0	11	20	156	5.08

	VIT A (IU)	VIT C (mg)	CAL (mg)	MAG (mg)	PHOS (mg)	ZINC (mg)
Round, bottom round, lean and fat, choice, braised (3 oz.)	0	0	5	19	208	4.17
Round, tip round, lean and fat, choice, roasted (3 oz.)	0	0	5	20	189	5.43
T-bone steak, short loin, all grades, broiled (3 oz.)	0	0	7	20	159	3.83
T-bone steak, short loin, choice, broiled (3 oz.)	0	0	7	20	156	3.78
T-bone steak, short loin, lean and fat, choice, broiled (3 oz.)	0	0	6	21	168	4.11
T-bone steak, short loin, lean, choice, broiled (3 oz.)	0	0	5	24	183	4.51
Tenderloin, lean and fat, choice, broiled (3 oz.)	0	0	7	22	178	4.11
Top sirloin, lean and fat, choice, broiled (3 oz.)	0	0	9	24	187	4.93

Game Meat

Beefalo, composite of cuts, roasted (3 oz.)	0	8	20	213	390	5.44
Bison, roasted (3 oz.)	0	0	7	22	178	3.13
Buffalo, roasted (3 oz.)	0	0	13	28	187	2.16
Rabbit, composite of cuts, roasted (3 oz.)	0	0	16	18	224	1.93

Lamb

Ground, broiled (3 oz.)	0	0	19	20	171	3.97

	VIT A (IU)	VIT C (mg)	CAL (mg)	MAG (mg)	PHOS (mg)	ZINC (mg)
Leg, domestic, sirloin half, lean and fat, choice, roasted (3 oz.)	0	0	9	19	156	3.51
Loin, domestic, lean only, choice, broiled (3 oz.)	0	0	16	24	192	3.51
Liver, braised (3 oz.)	21,203	3	7	19	357	6.71

Luncheon Meats

	VIT A (IU)	VIT C (mg)	CAL (mg)	MAG (mg)	PHOS (mg)	ZINC (mg)
Beef, thin sliced (5 slices)	0	0	2	4	35	0.84
Bologna, beef (1 slice)	0	0	3	3	20	0.5
Bologna, turkey (2 slices)	0	0	48	8	74	0.99
Ham, extra lean, 5% fat (1 slice)	0	0	2	5	62	0.55
Ham, regular, 11% fat (1 slice)	0	0	2	5	70	0.61
Pastrami, beef, cured (100 g)	0	0	9	18	150	4.26
Pastrami, turkey (2 slices)	0	0	5	8	113	1.23
Salami						
Beef, cooked (1 slice)	0	0	2	3	26	0.5
Beef, beer, beerwurst (1 slice)	0	0	2	3	22	0.56
Pork, beer, beerwurst (1 slice)	0	0	2	3	24	0.4
Pork, beef, dry or hard (1 slice)	0	0	1	2	14	0.32
Turkey, cooked (2 slices)	0	0	11	9	60	1.03

Pork

	VIT A (IU)	VIT C (mg)	CAL (mg)	MAG (mg)	PHOS (mg)	ZINC (mg)
Bacon, Canadian-style, grilled (2 slices)	0	0	5	10	138	0.79

	VIT A (IU)	VIT C (mg)	CAL (mg)	MAG (mg)	PHOS (mg)	ZINC (mg)
Bacon, cured, cooked, broiled, pan-fried, or roasted (3 med. slices)	0	0	2	5	64	0.62
Ham						
Cured, boneless, extra lean 5% fat (3 oz.)	0	0	7	12	167	2.45
Cured, extra lean, 4% fat, canned, roasted (3 oz.)	0	0	5	18	178	1.9
Patties, grilled (1 patty)	0	0	5	6	60	1.13
Steak, cured, boneless, extra lean (1 slice)	0	18	2	11	147	1.15

Sausage

	VIT A (IU)	VIT C (mg)	CAL (mg)	MAG (mg)	PHOS (mg)	ZINC (mg)
Bockwurst, pork, veal, uncooked (1 link)	15	0	10	12	95	1.01
Chorizo, pork and beef (1 link)	0	0	5	11	90	2.05
Frankfurter, beef (1 frankfurter)	0	0	9	1	39	0.98
Frankfurter, beef and pork (1 frankfurter)	0	0	5	5	39	0.83
Frankfurter, turkey (1 frankfurter)	0	0	48	6	60	1.4
Keilbasa, kolbassy, pork, beef, nonfat dry milk added (1 slice)	0	0	11	4	39	0.53
Link, smoked, pork (1 link)	0	1	20	13	110	1.92
Link, smoked, pork and beef, nonfat dry milk added (1 link)	0	0	28	11	93	1.33

Veal	VIT A (IU)	VIT C (mg)	CAL (mg)	MAG (mg)	PHOS (mg)	ZINC (mg)
Ground, broiled (3 oz.)	0	0	15	20	185	3.29
Leg, top round, lean and fat, braised (100 g)	0	0	8	29	249	3.96
Loin, lean and fat, braised (3 oz.)	0	0	24	20	187	3.09
Sirloin, lean only, braised (3 oz.)	0	0	16	25	220	4.04

Vegetarian, Meatless

	VIT A (IU)	VIT C (mg)	CAL (mg)	MAG (mg)	PHOS (mg)	ZINC (mg)
Bacon (1 strip)	4	0	1	1	4	0.02
Breakfast Patties, Morningstar Farms (1 patty)	0	0	18	1	106	0.37
Burgers, meatless						
Black Bean, spicy, Morningstar Farms (1 patty)	139	0	56	44	150	0.93
Crumbles, Morningstar Farms (1 cup)	0	0	79	2	174	1.64
Garden Vege Patties, Morningstar Farms (1 patty)	766	0	48	30	124	0.58
Harvest Burgers, Green Giant (⅔ cup)	0	0	100	*	*	4.5
Vegan, Morningstar Farms (1 patty)	0	0	87	16	181	0.75
Veggie Burgers, Yves (1 patty)	100	0	60	*	*	*
Deli slices, Veggie, Yves (3.5 slices)	0	0	30	*	*	*
Franks, Deli, Morningstar Farms (1 serving)	0	0	17	4	42	0.38
Sausage, meatless (1 patty)	243	0	24	14	86	0.56

	VIT A (IU)	VIT C (mg)	CAL (mg)	MAG (mg)	PHOS (mg)	ZINC (mg)
Tofu Crumbles, Vegetarian Hamburgers, Marjon (2½ oz.)	0	0	60	*	*	*
Wieners, Veggie, Yves (1 link)	0	0	20	*	*	*

MILK, CREAM, AND YOGURT

Milk

	VIT A (IU)	VIT C (mg)	CAL (mg)	MAG (mg)	PHOS (mg)	ZINC (mg)
1%, protein fortified, with added vitamin A (1 cup)	499	3	349	39	273	1.11
1%, with added nonfat solids and vitamin A (1 cup)	500	3	313	35	245	0.98
2%, protein fortified, with added vitamin A (1 cup)	500	3	352	40	276	1.11
2%, with added nonfat milk solids and vitamin A (1 cup)	500	3	313	35	245	0.98
3.3%, whole (1 cup)	307	2	291	33	228	0.93
Buttermilk, dried (1 tbsp.)	14	0	77	7	61	0.26
Buttermilk, fluid, cultured, from skim milk (1 cup)	81	2	285	27	219	1.03
CalciMilk, nonfat, A & D added (1 cup)	500	0	500	*	*	*
Chocolate beverage, hot cocoa, homemade (1 cup)	515	3	315	70	293	1.48

	VIT A (IU)	VIT C (mg)	CAL (mg)	MAG (mg)	PHOS (mg)	ZINC (mg)
Chocolate dairy drink mix, with aspartame, prepared with water (1 pkg., ½ cup water, 3 ice cubes)	120	0	94	23	89	0.4
Chocolate drink, fluid, commercial, 1% (1 cup)	500	2	287	33	257	1.03
Chocolate drink, fluid, commercial, 2% (1 cup)	500	2	284	33	254	1.03
Chocolate drink, fluid, commercial, whole (1 cup)	303	2	280	33	251	1.03
Condensed, sweetened, canned (1 cup)	1004	8	868	79	775	2.88
Dry, skim, nonfat solids, instant, with added vitamin A (⅓ cup)	545	1	283	27	227	1.01
Dry, skim, nonfat solids, regular, with added vitamin A (1 cup)	659	2	377	33	291	1.22
Dry, whole (¼ cup)	295	3	292	27	248	1.07
Dairy drink, chocolate, reduced-calorie, with aspartame, powder, prepared with water (6 oz.)	245	0	192	47	182	0.82
Evaporated, skim, canned (1 cup)	1004	3	741	69	499	2.3
Evaporated, whole, with added vitamin A (½ cup)	500	2	329	31	255	0.97
Evaporated, whole, without added vitamin A (1 cup)	612	5	657	61	510	1.94

	VIT A (IU)	VIT C (mg)	CAL (mg)	MAG (mg)	PHOS (mg)	ZINC (mg)
Goat, fluid (1 cup)	451	3	326	34	270	0.73
Lactose-free (1 cup)	500	*	300	*	*	*
Lactose-reduced (1 cup)	*	*	300	*	*	*
Lactose-reduced, calcium-fortified (1 cup)	*	*	500	*	*	*
Parmalat, whole, long life (½ pint)	300	3	300	*	*	*
Rice Dream, rice beverage, Imagine Foods (1 cup)	500	0	300	*	*	*
Shake, chocolate, thick (10.6 oz.)	258	0	396	48	378	1.44
Shake, vanilla, thick (11 oz.)	357	0	457	37	361	1.22
Skim, protein fortified, with added vitamin A (1 cup)	499	3	352	40	275	1.11
Skim, with added nonfat milk solids and vitamin A (1 cup)	500	3	316	36	255	1
Soy milk (1 cup)	78	0	10	47	120	0.56
Soy Moo, fat-free, nondairy, lactose-free (1 cup)	0	0	400	*	*	*
Whole, low-sodium (1 cup)	317	2	246	12	209	0.93
Vitamite, 2% fat, nondairy, 100% lactose-free, added calcium and milk protein (1 cup)	500	0	200	*	100	*

Cream

	VIT A (IU)	VIT C (mg)	CAL (mg)	MAG (mg)	PHOS (mg)	ZINC (mg)
Cream topping, whipped, pressurized (1 tbsp.)	27	0	3	0	3	0.01

	VIT A (IU)	VIT C (mg)	CAL (mg)	MAG (mg)	PHOS (mg)	ZINC (mg)
Half and half (1 oz.)	131	0	32	3	29	0.15
Heavy, whipping, fluid (1 oz.)	438	0	19	2	19	0.07
Light, coffee or table, fluid (1 oz.)	216	0	29	3	24	0.08
Light, whipping, fluid (1 tbsp.)	169	0	10	1	9	0.04
Sour, cultured (1 tbsp.)	95	0	14	1	10	0.03
Sour dressing, nonbutterfat, cultured, filled cream-type (1 tbsp.)	1	0	14	1	11	0.04
Sour, half and half, cultured (1 tbsp.)	68	0	16	2	14	0.08
Sour, imitation, cultured (1 oz.)	0	0	1	2	13	0.34

Yogurt

	VIT A (IU)	VIT C (mg)	CAL (mg)	MAG (mg)	PHOS (mg)	ZINC (mg)
Coffee, low-fat, 11 g protein per 1 cup (1 cup)	132	2	420	40	330	2.03
Fruit, low-fat, 9 g protein per 1 cup (1 cup)	120	2	339	33	266	1.64
Fruit, low-fat, 10 g protein per 1 cup (1 cup)	104	2	345	33	271	1.68
Fruit, low-fat, 11 g protein per 1 cup (1 cup)	136	2	383	37	301	1.86
Frozen, chocolate, soft-serve (1/2 cup)	115	0	106	19	100	0.35
Frozen, vanilla, soft-serve (1/2 cup)	153	1	103	10	93	0.3
Plain, fat-free (1 cup)	0	0	400	*	*	*
Plain, low-fat, 12 g protein per 1 cup (1 cup)	162	2	447	43	352	2.18

	VIT A (IU)	VIT C (mg)	CAL (mg)	MAG (mg)	PHOS (mg)	ZINC (mg)
Plain, skim milk, 13 g protein per 1 cup (1 cup)	17	2	488	47	383	2.38
Plain, whole milk, 8 g protein per 1 cup (1 cup)	301	1	296	28	233	1.45

MISCELLANEOUS

Condiments

Catsup (1 tbsp.)	152	2	3	3	6	0.04
Catsup, low-sodium (1 tbsp.)	152	2	3	3	6	0.04
Mayonnaise (1 tbsp.)	32	0	2	*	4	*
Mustard, yellow (1 tbsp.)	0	*	4	*	4	*
Pepper sauce, hot (¼ tsp.)	4	1	0	0	0	0
Pickle, cucumber, dill (1 spear)	99	1	3	3	6	0.04
Pickle, cucumber, sweet (1 pickle)	3	0	1	1	3	0.02
Pickle relish						
Hamburger (1 tbsp.)	40	0	1	1	3	0.02
Hot dog (1 tbsp.)	25	0	1	3	6	0.03
Sweet (1 tbsp.)	23	0	1	1	2	0.02
Soy sauce (1 tbsp.)	0	0	3	6	20	0.07
Soy sauce, made from soy and wheat (shoyu), low-sodium (1 tbsp.)	0	0	3	6	20	0.07
Soy sauce, made from soy, tamari (1 tbsp.)	0	0	4	7	23	0.08
Tahini, sesame butter (1 oz.)	19	0	121	27	208	1.31
Tabasco, pepper, ready-to-serve (¼ tsp.)	20	0	0	0	0	0

	VIT A (IU)	VIT C (mg)	CAL (mg)	MAG (mg)	PHOS (mg)	ZINC (mg)
Tartar sauce (1 tbsp.)	30	*	3	*	4	*
Teriyaki (1 tbsp.)	0	0	4	11	28	0.02
Vinegar, cidar (1 tbsp.)	0	0	1	*	1	*

Leavening Agents

	VIT A (IU)	VIT C (mg)	CAL (mg)	MAG (mg)	PHOS (mg)	ZINC (mg)
Baking powder, double-acting, low-sodium (1 tsp.)	0	0	216	1	343	0.03
Baking powder, double-acting, sodium and aluminum (1 tsp.)	0	0	270	1	100	0
Baking powder, double-acting, straight phosphate (1 tsp.)	0	0	338	2	456	0

Spices

	VIT A (IU)	VIT C (mg)	CAL (mg)	MAG (mg)	PHOS (mg)	ZINC (mg)
Allspice, ground (1 tsp.)	10	1	13	3	2	0.02
Anise seed (1 tsp.)	7	0	14	4	9	0.11
Basil, fresh (2 tbsp.)	205	1	8	4	4	0.05
Basil, ground (1 tsp.)	131	1	30	6	7	0.08
Bay leaf, crumbled (1 tsp.)	37	0	5	1	1	0.02
Caraway seed (1 tsp.)	8	0	15	5	12	0.12
Cardamon, ground (1 tsp.)	0	0	8	5	4	0.15
Celery seed (1 tsp.)	1	0	35	9	11	0.14
Chervil, dried (1 tsp.)	35	0	8	1	3	0.05
Chili powder (1 tsp.)	908	2	7	4	8	0.07
Cilantro (1 oz.)	256	3	*	*	*	*
Cinnamon, ground (1 tsp.)	6	1	28	1	1	0.05
Cloves, ground (1 tsp.)	11	2	14	6	2	0.02
Coriander leaf, dried (1 tsp.)	35	3	8	4	3	0.03
Coriander seed (1 tsp.)	0	0	13	6	7	0.09

	VIT A (IU)	VIT C (mg)	CAL (mg)	MAG (mg)	PHOS (mg)	ZINC (mg)
Cumin seed (1 tsp.)	27	0	20	8	10	0.1
Curry powder (1 tsp.)	20	0	10	5	7	0.08
Dill seed (1 tsp.)	1	0	32	5	6	0.11
Dill weed, dried (1 tsp.)	59	1	18	5	5	0.03
Dill weed, fresh (10 sprigs)	144	2	5	1	1	0.02
Fennel seed (1 tsp.)	3	0	24	8	10	0.07
Fenugreek seed (1 tsp.)	2	0	7	7	11	0.09
Garlic powder (1 tsp.)	0	1	2	2	12	0.07
Ginger, ground (1 tsp.)	3	0	2	3	3	0.09
Mace, ground (1 tsp.)	14	0	4	3	2	0.04
Marjoram, dried (1 tsp.)	48	0	12	2	2	0.02
Mustard, seed, yellow (1 tsp.)	2	0	17	10	28	0.19
Nutmeg, ground (1 tsp.)	2	0	4	4	5	0.05
Onion powder (1 tsp.)	0	0	8	3	7	0.05
Oregano, ground (1 tsp.)	104	1	24	4	3	0.07
Parsley, dried (1 tsp.)	70	0	4	1	1	0.01
Pepper, black (1 tsp.)	4	0	9	4	4	0.03
Pepper, red or cayenne (1 tsp.)	749	1	3	3	5	0.05
Pepper, white (1 tsp.)	0	1	6	2	4	0.03
Poppy seed (1 tsp.)	0	0	41	9	24	0.29
Poultry seasoning (1 tsp.)	40	0	15	3	3	0.05
Pumpkin pie spice (1 tsp.)	4	0	12	2	2	0.04
Rosemary, dried (1 tsp.)	38	1	15	3	1	0.04
Saffron (1 tsp.)	4	1	1	2	2	0.01
Sage, ground (1 tsp.)	41	0	12	3	1	0.03
Salt, table (1 tsp.)	0	0	1	0	0	0.01
Savory, ground (1 tsp.)	72	1	30	5	2	0.06
Thyme, fresh (1 tsp.)	38	1	3	1	1	0.01
Thyme, ground (1 tsp.)	53	1	26	3	3	0.09
Tumeric, ground (1 tsp.)	0	1	4	4	6	0.1

Sugars and syrups	VIT A (IU)	VIT C (mg)	CAL (mg)	MAG (mg)	PHOS (mg)	ZINC (mg)
Sugar						
Brown (1 tsp.)	0	0	3	1	1	0.01
Granulated (1 tsp.)	0	0	0	0	0	0
Maple (1 oz.)	7	0	26	5	1	1.72
Powdered (1 tsp.)	0	0	0	0	0	0
Syrups						
Corn, dark (1 tbsp.)	0	0	4	2	2	0.01
Corn, table blends, refined and sugar (1 tbsp.)	0	0	5	2	2	0.01
Molasses, blackstrap (1 tbsp.)	0	0	172	43	8	0.02
Pancake, table blend (1 tbsp.)	0	0	0	0	2	0.01
Pancake, table blend, reduced-calorie (1 oz.)	0	0	0	0	12	0.01
Syrups, flavored						
Chocolate, with added nutrients, prepared with milk (1 cup)	1126	2	292	32	229	0.92
Strawberry-flavor beverage mix prepared with milk (1 cup)	309	2	293	32	229	0.93

Thickening Agent

Cornstarch (1 cup)	0	0	3	4	17	0.07

NUTS, SEEDS, AND BUTTERS

Nuts

Almonds						
Honey roasted (1 oz.)	0	0	75	68	113	0.74

	VIT A (IU)	VIT C (mg)	CAL (mg)	MAG (mg)	PHOS (mg)	ZINC (mg)
Dried, blanched (1 oz.)	0	0	70	81	151	0.9
Dry roasted, unblanched (1 oz.)	0	0	80	86	155	1.39
Oil roasted, blanched (1 oz.)	0	0	55	82	164	0.4
Toasted, unblanched (1 oz.)	0	0	80	87	156	1.4
Butternuts, dried (1 oz.)	35	1	15	67	126	0.89
Cashew nuts, dry-roasted (1 oz.)	0	0	13	74	139	1.59
Chestnuts, Chinese, roasted (1 oz.)	1	11	5	26	29	0.26
Coconut meat, raw, shredded (1 cup)	0	3	11	26	90	0.88
Filberts, dried, unblanched (1 oz.)	19	0	53	81	89	0.68
Filberts, dry-roasted, unblanched (1 oz.)	0	0	55	84	92	0.71
Ginkgo, canned (1 oz.)	96	3	1	5	15	0.06
Ginkgo, dried (1 oz.)	309	8	6	15	76	0.19
Macadamia, dried (1 oz.)	0	0	20	33	39	0.49
Macadamia, oil-roasted (1 oz.)	3	0	13	33	57	0.31
Mixed nuts, dry-roasted, with peanuts (1 oz.)	4	0	20	64	123	1.08
Peanuts, all types, raw (1 oz.)	0	0	26	48	107	0.93
Pecans, dried (1 oz.)	36	1	10	36	83	1.55
Pine, dried (10 kernels)	0	0	0	2	0	0.04
Pine, pignolia, dried (1 oz.)	8	1	7	66	144	1.21
Pistachio, dried (1 oz.)	66	2	38	45	143	0.38
Pistachio, dry-roasted (1 oz.)	67	2	20	37	135	0.39
Soy, roasted (1 oz.)	0	0	60	*	*	*

	VIT A (IU)	VIT C (mg)	CAL (mg)	MAG (mg)	PHOS (mg)	ZINC (mg)
Walnuts, black, dried (1 oz.)	84	1	16	57	132	0.97
Walnuts, English or Persian dried (1 oz.)	35	1	27	48	90	0.77
Wheat based, unflavored (1 oz.)	0	0	7	16	105	0.83
Seeds						
Alfalfa, sprouted, raw (1 cup)	51	3	11	9	23	0.3
Breadfruit, boiled (1 oz.)	68	2	17	4	35	0.24
Breadfruit, raw (1 oz.)	73	2	10	15	50	0.27
Breadnut tree seeds, dried (1 oz.)	61	13	27	33	51	0.54
Breadnut tree seeds, raw (1 oz., 8–14 seeds)	70	8	28	19	19	0.32
Pumpkin kernels, roasted (1 oz.)	108	1	12	152	333	2.11
Pumpkin and squash seed kernels, roasted, with salt (1 oz.)	108	1	12	152	333	2.11
Pumpkin and squash seed kernels, roasted, with salt (1 cup)	862	4	98	1212	2660	16.9
Sesame, whole, dried (1 tbsp.)	1	0	88	32	57	0.7
Sesame, whole, roasted and toasted (1 oz.)	3	0	280	101	181	2.03
Soybeans, mature, roasted (½ cup)	172	2	119	125	312	2.7
Squash, kernels, roasted (1 oz.)	108	1	12	151	332	2.11

	VIT A (IU)	VIT C (mg)	CAL (mg)	MAG (mg)	PHOS (mg)	ZINC (mg)
Sunflower seeds						
Dried (½ cup)	36	1	134	255	507	3.6
Dry-roasted (1 oz.)	0	0	20	37	327	1.5
Roasted (½ cup)	*	*	40	220	500	*
Roasted, reduced-sodium (½ cup)	*	*	40	220	500	*
Roasted, reduced-sodium (1 cup)	*	*	80	440	1000	*
Watermelon kernels, dried (1 oz.)	0	0	15	146	214	2.9
Butters						
Almond, honey and cinnamon (1 tbsp.)	0	0	43	48	83	0.48
Almond, plain (1 tbsp.)	0	0	43	49	84	0.49
Almond paste (1 oz.)	0	<1	65	73	127	0.73
Apple butter (1 tbsp.)	0	*	1	0	1	0.01
Cashew, plain (1 tbsp.)	0	0	7	41	73	0.83
Peanut, chunk style (2 tbsp.)	0	0	13	51	101	0.89
Peanut, Plus Vitamins and Minerals (2 tbsp.)	1250	*	*	87	*	3
Peanut, reduced-fat (2 tbsp.)	0	0	0	45	0	0.9
Peanut, smooth style (2 tbsp.)	0	0	12	51	118	0.93
Sesame, paste (1 tbsp.)	8	0	154	58	105	1.17
Sesame, tahini, from roasted and toasted kernels (1 tbsp.)	10	0	64	14	110	0.69
Sunflower seed (1 tbsp.)	8	0	20	59	118	0.85

PASTA, NOODLES, AND RICE	VIT A (IU)	VIT C (mg)	CAL (mg)	MAG (mg)	PHOS (mg)	ZINC (mg)
Pasta						
Corn, cooked (1 cup)	80	0	1	50	106	0.88
Corn, dry (2 oz.)	97	0	2	68	144	1.02
Couscous, cooked (1 cup)	0	0	13	13	35	0.41
Homemade, with egg, cooked (2 oz.)	33	0	6	8	30	0.25
Homemade, without egg, cooked (2 oz.)	0	0	3	8	23	0.21
Plain, fresh-refrigerated, as purchased (4.5 oz.)	60	0	19	59	209	1.56
Plain, fresh-refrigerated, cooked (2 oz.)	11	0	3	10	36	0.32
Spaghetti						
Protein-fortified, dry pasta, enriched (2 oz.)	0	0	22	37	93	1.02
Spinach pasta, cooked (1 cup)	213	0	42	87	151	1.51
Spinach, fresh-refrigerated, as purchased (4.5 oz.)	308	0	55	81	189	1.79
Spinach pasta, fresh-refrigerated, cooked (2 oz.)	59	0	10	14	33	0.36
Whole wheat, dry pasta (2 oz.)	0	0	23	82	147	1.35
Noodles						
Chinese, chow mein (1.5 oz.)	37	0	9	22	69	0.6

	VIT A (IU)	VIT C (mg)	CAL (mg)	MAG (mg)	PHOS (mg)	ZINC (mg)
Egg, enriched, cooked (1 cup)	32	0	19	30	110	0.99
Egg, spinach, enriched, cooked (1 cup)	165	0	30	38	91	1.01
Macaroni, protein-fortified, enriched, cooked (½ cup)	0	0	6	17	29	0.29
Macaroni, vegetable, enriched, cooked (1 cup)	71	0	15	26	67	0.59
Macaroni, whole-wheat, dry (1 cup)	0	0	42	150	271	2.49
Protein-fortified, enriched, dry (2 oz.)	0	0	22	37	93	1.02
Soba, Japanese, cooked (1 cup)	0	0	5	10	29	0.14
Somen, Japanese, cooked (1 cup)	0	0	14	4	48	0.39
Whole wheat, elbow, dry (1 cup)	0	0	23	82	147	1.35
Whole wheat, spiral, dry (1 cup)	0	0	42	150	271	2.49

Rice *(see also* Grains)

	VIT A (IU)	VIT C (mg)	CAL (mg)	MAG (mg)	PHOS (mg)	ZINC (mg)
Brown, long-grained, cooked (1 cup)	0	0	20	84	162	1.23
White, glutinous, cooked (1 cup)	0	0	4	9	14	0.71
White, long-grained, parboiled, enriched, cooked (1 cup)	0	0	33	21	74	0.54
White, long-grained, precooked or instant, enriched, prepared (1 cup)	0	0	13	8	23	0.4

	VIT A (IU)	VIT C (mg)	CAL (mg)	MAG (mg)	PHOS (mg)	ZINC (mg)
White, long-grained, regular, cooked (1 cup)	0	0	16	19	68	0.77
White, with pasta, cooked (1 cup)	0	0	16	24	75	0.57
White, with pasta, dry (1 cup)	0	1	75	65	258	1.97
Wild, cooked (1 cup)	0	0	5	53	135	2.2

POULTRY

Chicken

Broilers or fryers, fried						
Breast, meat and skin, floured, bone removed (½ breast)	49	0	16	29	228	1.08
Dark meat, meat only (1 cup)	111	0	25	35	262	4.08
Giblets (1 cup)	17,297	13	26	36	415	0.09
Light meat, meat only (1 cup)	42	0	22	41	323	1.78
Broilers or fryers, roasted						
Back, meat only, bone and skin removed (½ back)	38	0	10	9	66	1.06
Breast, meat and skin, bone removed (½ breast)	91	0	14	27	210	1
Breast, meat only, bone and skin removed (½ breast)	18	0	13	25	196	0.86

	VIT A (IU)	VIT C (mg)	CAL (mg)	MAG (mg)	PHOS (mg)	ZINC (mg)
Dark meat, meat and skin, ready to cook chicken (1 lb.)	203	0	15	22	170	2.52
Dark meat, meat only (1 cup, chopped)	101	0	21	32	251	3.92
Drumstick, meat only, bone and skin removed (1 drumstick)	26	0	5	11	81	1.4
Light meat, meat only, chopped (1 cup)	41	0	21	38	302	1.72
Light meat, meat and skin, ready-to-cook (1 lb.)	87	0	12	20	158	0.97
Meat, skin, giblets and neck, ready-to-cook (1 lb.)	1304	1	31	47	373	4.43
Thigh, meat only (1 cup)	91	0	17	34	256	3.6
Cornish game hens, meat and skin (½ bird)	136	0.5	17	23	188	1.92
Cornish game hens, meat and skin (1 whole bird)	272	1	33	46	375	3.83
Frankfurter, chicken (1 frankfurter)	59	0	43	5	48	0.47
Liver, all classes, simmered (1 cup, chopped)	22,925	22	20	29	437	6.08

Meatless Poultry

Chicken, vegetarian, canned, Worthington (3 slices)	0	0	13	*	112	0.4

	VIT A (IU)	VIT C (mg)	CAL (mg)	MAG (mg)	PHOS (mg)	ZINC (mg)
Chicken, Vetetarian, frozen, Morningstar Farms (1 patty)	0	0	11	*	121	0.31
Chicken Nuggets, Vegetarian, Loma Linda (5 pieces)	0	0	41	*	*	0.43

Turkey

	VIT A (IU)	VIT C (mg)	CAL (mg)	MAG (mg)	PHOS (mg)	ZINC (mg)
Bologna (2 slices)	0	0	48	8	74	0.99
Breast (2 slices)	0	0	3	9	97	0.48
Breast, meat and skin, ready-to-cook (1 lb.)	0	0	24	30	235	2.27
Dark meat (1 cup, chopped)	0	0	45	34	286	6.24
Frankfurter, turkey (1 frankfurter)	0	0	48	6	60	1.4
Giblets, simmered (1 cup, chopped)	8752	3	19	25	296	5.34
Gizzard, simmered (1 cup, cooked)	268	2	22	28	186	6.03
Ground, cooked (1 patty, 4 oz. raw)	0	0	21	20	161	2.35
Ham, cured turkey thigh meat (2 slices)	0	0	6	9	108	1.67
Hen, young, meat only, roasted (1 cup, chopped)	0	0	35	36	297	4.24
Leg, meat and skin, roasted, bone removed (1 leg)	0	0	175	126	1087	23.31
Liver, simmered (1 cup, chopped)	17,613	3	15	21	381	4.33
Meat only, roasted (1 cup, chopped)	0	0	35	36	298	4.34

	VIT A (IU)	VIT C (mg)	CAL (mg)	MAG (mg)	PHOS (mg)	ZINC (mg)
Meat, skin, giblets, and neck, roasted, ready to cook (1 lb.)	598	0	68	62	520	8.19
Pastrami, turkey (2 slices)	0	0	5	8	113	1.23
Patties, turkey, breaded, battered, fried (1 patty)	35	0	13	14	254	1.35
Roll, turkey, light meat (2 slices)	0	0	23	9	104	0.89
Roll, turkey, dark meat (2 slices)	0	0	18	10	95	1.13
Salami, cooked, turkey (2 slices)	0	0	11	9	60	1.03

Game and Other Poultry

Duck

	VIT A (IU)	VIT C (mg)	CAL (mg)	MAG (mg)	PHOS (mg)	ZINC (mg)
Domesticated, meat only, roasted, ready-to-cook (1 lb.)	77	0	12	20	203	2.6
Domesticated, meat and skin, roasted, ready-to-cook (1 lb.)	363	0	19	28	270	3.22
Wild, breast, meat only, raw, skin removed (½ breast)	44	5	3	18	154	0.61

Goose

	VIT A (IU)	VIT C (mg)	CAL (mg)	MAG (mg)	PHOS (mg)	ZINC (mg)
Domesticated, meat only, roasted, ready-to-cook (1 lb.)	57	0	20	36	442	4.53
Domesticated, meat and skin, roasted, ready-to-cook (1 lb.)	132	0	24	41	508	4.93

	VIT A (IU)	VIT C (mg)	CAL (mg)	MAG (mg)	PHOS (mg)	ZINC (mg)
Pâté, goose liver, smoked, canned (1 oz.)	945	0	20	4	57	0.26

Pheasant

	VIT A (IU)	VIT C (mg)	CAL (mg)	MAG (mg)	PHOS (mg)	ZINC (mg)
Breast, meat only, raw, bone and skin removed (½ breast)	268	11	6	38	364	1.15
Meat only, raw, ready-to-cook (1 lb.)	538	20	42	65	750	3.16
Meat and skin, raw, ready-to-cook (1 lb.)	657	20	45	74	794	3.56
Quail, meat and skin, raw (1 oz.)	69	2	4	*	61	*

PREPARED FOODS

	VIT A (IU)	VIT C (mg)	CAL (mg)	MAG (mg)	PHOS (mg)	ZINC (mg)
Amaranth Dinner with Garden Vegetables, canned, Health Valley (7½ oz.)	*	*	40	*	*	*
Beans						
Plain or vegetarian (1 cup)	434	8	127	81	264	3.56
With franks, canned (1 cup)	399	6	124	73	269	4.84
With franks, frozen, Banquet (10¼ oz.)	4450	*	130	*	*	*
Baked, with pork and sweet sauce, canned (1 cup)	288	8	154	86	266	3.8
Beef, Extra Helping, frozen, Banquet (10¼ oz.)	4600	*	80	*	*	*

	VIT A (IU)	VIT C (mg)	CAL (mg)	MAG (mg)	PHOS (mg)	ZINC (mg)
Biscuit, Egg and Cheese, frozen, precooked, Sunny Fresh (1 serving)	205	0	101	3	50	0.3
Biscuit, egg and steak (1 biscuit)	705	0	138	25	225	2.8
Biscuit, Egg, Ham and Cheese, Sunny Fresh (1 serving)	213	0	106	4	54	0.33
Black Bean Dinner, with Garden Vegetables, Health Valley (7½ oz.)	4550	*	150	*	*	0.96
Brunswick Stew, homemade (1 cup)	400	*	30	*	*	1.67
Chicken and Dumplings, frozen, Banquet (9 oz.)	2950	*	50	*	*	*
Chicken in Cheese Sauce with Broccoli, frozen, Light and Elegant (8¾ oz.)	350	*	170	*	*	*
Chicken Piccatta with Rice, frozen, Prego (11 oz.)	850	*	80	*	*	*
Chicken with Broccoli, frozen, Light and Elegant (9½ oz.)	350	*	170	*	*	*
Chopped Beef, frozen, Banquet (11 oz.)	6400	*	60	*	*	*
Chili, Beans, Nestlé, Chef-Mate (1 cup)	3013	1	89	46	167	3.87
Chili, beans, canned (1 cup)	863	4	120	115	394	5.12
Corn pudding (⅔ cup)	411	5	67	25	95	0.84

	VIT A (IU)	VIT C (mg)	CAL (mg)	MAG (mg)	PHOS (mg)	ZINC (mg)
Enchilada Beef, frozen, Banquet (12 oz.)	350	*	170	*	*	*
Enchilada, cheese (1 enchilada)	300	9	150	*	*	*
Enchilada, black bean, vegetable (1 enchilada)	400	6	40	*	*	*
Garden Vegetable Lasagna, Campbell's, frozen (1 cup)	3500	3	450	*	*	*
Hash, corned beef (1 cup)	0	2	46	38	240	7.51
Hush puppy, prepared from recipe (1 hush puppy)	31	0	61	5	42	0.15
Hummus (1 cup)	61	19	124	71	275	2.7
Lasagna Alfredo, Weight Watcher's (½ cup)	200	6	250	*	*	*
Florentine, frozen, Light and Elegant (12 oz.)	1300	*	70	*	*	*
Meat Sauce, frozen, Banquet (11¼ oz.)	3850	*	230	*	*	*
Lentil Dinner, with Garden Vegetable, canned, Health Valley (7½ oz.)	5200	*	70	*	*	0.64
Macaroni and cheese						
Canned, Franco-American (7½ oz.)	550	*	170	*	*	*
Kraft (¾ cup)	350	*	100	*	*	1.28
Nestlé, Chef-Mate (1 cup)	210	0	202	33	251	1.57
Manicotti with 3 Cheeses, Healthy Choice, frozen (1 serving)	750	*	350	*	*	*

	VIT A (IU)	VIT C (mg)	CAL (mg)	MAG (mg)	PHOS (mg)	ZINC (mg)
Mexican Style Dinner, Extra Helping, Banquet (21¼ oz.)	1200	*	340	*	*	*
Muffins, wheat bran, prepared from recipe, with whole milk (1 muffin)	459	5	106	45	163	1.57
Onion rings, breaded, frozen (7 rings)	158	1	22	13	57	0.29
Pasta Primavera Style, frozen, Bird's Eye (½ cup)	4050	*	80	*	*	0.64
Peas and Potatoes with Cream Sauce, Bird's Eye (½ cup)	500	*	40	*	*	0.48
Pizza, cheese (1 slice)	382	1	117	16	113	0.81
Pizza, cheese, meat, and vegetables (1 slice)	524	2	101	18	131	1.11
Pizza sauce, ready-to-serve (¼ cup)	420	7	34	13	32	0.16
Poi, taro root (1 cup)	48	10	38	58	94	0.53
Potatoes						
Au gratin, dry mix, prepared with water, whole milk, and butter (⅙ of 5.5 oz. package)	292	4	114	21	130	0.33
Au gratin, home-prepared from recipe using butter (1 cup)	647	24	292	49	277	1.69
Cream and Chives, baked, frozen, Pillsbury (1 potato)	400	*	40	*	*	*

	VIT A (IU)	VIT C (mg)	CAL (mg)	MAG (mg)	PHOS (mg)	ZINC (mg)
French fried, home-prepared, heated in oven (10 strips)	0	5	4	11	41	0.2
Hash brown, frozen, butter sauce, prepared (100 g)	111	4	33	15	38	0.33
Hash brown, frozen, plain, prepared (1 oval patty)	0	2	4	5	21	0.09
Hash brown, home-prepared (1 cup)	0	9	13	31	66	0.47
Mashed, dehydrated, granules with milk, dry form (1 cup)	120	32	284	148	474	2.4
Mashed, flakes, without milk, dry (1 cup)	0	40	12	31	74	0.33
Mashed, home-prepared, whole milk and margarine added (1 cup)	355	13	55	38	97	0.57
Mashed, home-prepared, whole milk, butter (1 cup)	355	13	55	38	97	0.57
Potato pancakes, home-prepared (1 pancake)	109	17	18	25	84	0.63
Potato salad (1/3 cup)	95	1	13	8	53	0.19
Scalloped, dry mix, prepared with water, whole milk, and butter (1/6 of 5.5 oz. package)	203	5	49	19	77	0.34
Scalloped, home-prepared with butter (1/2 cup)	166	13	70	24	77	0.49

	VIT A (IU)	VIT C (mg)	CAL (mg)	MAG (mg)	PHOS (mg)	ZINC (mg)
Scalloped, home-prepared with butter (1 cup)	331	26	140	47	154	0.98
Ravioli with Meat, Sausage and Peppers, Prego Plus (1 cup)	2000	*	80	*	*	*
Refried beans, canned (½ cup)	*	8	44	42	109	1.48
Refried beans, canned (1 cup)	*	15	88	83	217	2.95
Relish, cranberry-orange, canned (½ cup)	87	25	15	11	11	*
Relish, cranberry-orange, canned (1 cup)	193	50	30	11	22	*
Rice						
Black-Eyed Peas and Rice, Zatarain, prepared (½ cup)	*	0	40	*	*	*
Dirty Rice Mix, Zatarain, prepared (1 cup)	100	1	40	*	*	*
Pinto Beans and Rice, Uncle Ben's, prepared (1 cup)	400	3	40	*	*	*
Wild Rice & Mushroom Stuffing Mix, Pepperidge Farm, prepared (⅔ cup)	*	6	40	*	*	*
Rosetto, cheese stuffed shells (2 pieces)	400	*	200	*	*	*

	VIT A (IU)	VIT C (mg)	CAL (mg)	MAG (mg)	PHOS (mg)	ZINC (mg)
Shrimp Creole, with Rice and Peppers, Light and Elegant (10 oz.)	2200	*	60	*	*	*
Spaghetti with Meat Sauce, canned, Prego (12½ oz.)	1300	*	40	*	*	*
Spanish Rice, canned, Van Camp (1 cup)	1150	*	30	*	*	*
Spinach soufflé (1 cup)	3461	3	230	38	231	1.29
Stew, Beef, Nestlé, Chef-Mate (1 cup)	3107	3	63	35	159	2.5
Stuffing, corn bread, prepared (½ cup)	44	1	22	12	32	0.21
Stuffing, prepared (½ cup)	*	*	28	11	40	0.26
Tomato Pasta Florentine, frozen, Campbell's (½ cup)	750	6	80	*	*	*
Tuna Pot Pie, frozen, Banquet (1 cup)	150	*	50	*	*	*
Turkey Pot Pie, frozen, Banquet (1 cup)	150	*	40	*	*	*
Turkey Tetrazzini, frozen, Banquet (10 oz.)	350	*	120	*	*	*
Veal Parmigiana, frozen, Banquet (11 oz.)	750	*	100	*	*	*
Taco mix (3 tbsp.)	122	0	20	*	*	0.32

Vegetarian entrées

	VIT A (IU)	VIT C (mg)	CAL (mg)	MAG (mg)	PHOS (mg)	ZINC (mg)
Beans, plain or vegetarian (1 cup)	434	8	127	81	264	3.56
Burgers						
Black Bean Burgers, spicy, Morningstar Farms (1 patty)	0	0	40	*	*	*

	VIT A (IU)	VIT C (mg)	CAL (mg)	MAG (mg)	PHOS (mg)	ZINC (mg)
California Veggie Burger, Organic Vegetables, Amy's (1 burger)	1500	3	20	*	*	*
Garden Vege Patties, Morningstar Farms (1 patty)	3	0	40	*	*	*
Egg Roll, Vegetarian, frozen, Worthington (3 oz. roll)	0	0	15	*	70	0.31
Falafel (2¼" patty)	2	*	9	14	33	0.26
Hummus, commercially prepared (½ cup)	31	10	62	36	138	1.35
Hummus, prepared from recipe (1 cup)	61	19	124	71	275	2.7
Lentil-Rice Loaf, Natural Touch (3.2 oz. slice)	775	0	21	*	213	1.04
Nine-Bean Loaf, Natural Touch (1" slice, 3 oz.)	1509	1	27	*	*	0.88
Savory Dinner Loaf, Loma Linda (⅓ cup)	0	0	23	*	*	0.38
Spinach Feta Pocketfuls, Amy's (1 serving)	2250	5	250	*	*	*
Tempeh (½ cup)	569	0	77	58	171	1.5
Vegetable Lasagna, Amy's (1 container)	2500	21	200	*	*	*
Vegetable Pot Pie, Amy's (1 container)	2250	5	100	*	*	*
Veggie Loaf, Mashed potatoes and Vegetables, Amy's (1 container)	2250	36	40	*	*	*

SALADS	VIT A (IU)	VIT C (mg)	CAL (mg)	MAG (mg)	PHOS (mg)	ZINC (mg)
Coleslaw (¾ cup)	338	8	34	9	36	0.2
Crab (1 serving)	30	2	38	26	*	*
Chef (1 serving)	2997	21	150	*	*	*
Carrot and raisin, homemade (1 serving)	3663	12	96	42	*	*
Tuna, with bread, lettuce, and oil (9 oz.)	188	4	74	79	219	*
Vegetable salads						
With egg and cheese, without dressing (1½ cups)	822	10	100	24	132	1
With chicken, without dressing (1½ cups)	935	17	37	33	170	0.89
With shrimp, without dressing (1½ cups)	791	9	59	38	161	1.27
Without dressing (1½ cups)	2352	48	27	23	81	0.44
Potato, homemade (1 cup)	500	*	40	*	*	0.61
Taco (1½ cups)	588	4	192	52	143	2.69
Taboule wheat salad mix (1 tbsp.)	100	0	40	*	*	*

SALAD DRESSINGS

	VIT A (IU)	VIT C (mg)	CAL (mg)	MAG (mg)	PHOS (mg)	ZINC (mg)
Blue or Roquefort cheese, regular (1 tbsp.)	32	0	12	0	11	0.04
French, diet, low-fat, 5 calories per teaspoon (1 tbsp.)	212	0	2	0	2	0.03
French, regular (1 tbsp.)	203	0	2	0	2	0.01

	VIT A (IU)	VIT C (mg)	CAL (mg)	MAG (mg)	PHOS (mg)	ZINC (mg)
Italian, diet, 2 calories per teaspoon (1 tbsp.)	0	0	0	0	1	0.02
Italian, diet, commercial (packet)	0	0	1	0	3	0.07
Italian, regular (1 tbsp.)	12	0	2	0	1	0.02
Oil and Vinegar, prepared by recipe (1 tbsp.)	0	0	0	0	*	*
Sesame seed (1 tbsp.)	106	0	3	0	6	0.02
Russian (1 tbsp.)	106	1	3	0	6	0.07
Thousand island, commercial (1 tbsp.)	50	0	2	0	3	0.02
Thousand island, diet, 10 calories per teaspoon (1 tbsp.)	49	0	2	0	3	0.02
Thousand island, regular (1 tbsp.)	50	0	2	0	3	0.02

SEAFOOD

	VIT A (IU)	VIT C (mg)	CAL (mg)	MAG (mg)	PHOS (mg)	ZINC (mg)
Anchovy, European, canned in oil, drained (1 can, 2 oz.)	32	0	104	31	113	1.1
Anchovy, European, raw (3 oz.)	43	0	125	35	148	1.46
Bass, fresh water, mixed species, cooked, dry heat (3 oz.)	98	2	88	32	218	0.71
Bass, fresh water, mixed species, raw (3 oz.)	85	2	68	26	170	0.55
Bluefish, cooked, dry heat (3 oz.)	390	0	8	36	247	0.88

	VIT A (IU)	VIT C (mg)	CAL (mg)	MAG (mg)	PHOS (mg)	ZINC (mg)
Burbot, cooked, dry heat (3 oz.)	15	0	54	35	218	0.83
Butterfish, cooked, dry heat (3 oz.)	93	0	24	27	262	0.84
Catfish, channel, breaded, fried (1 fillet)	24	0	38	24	188	0.75
Catfish, channel, farmed, cooked, dry heat (3 oz.)	43	1	8	22	208	0.89
Catfish, channel, wild, cooked, dry heat (3 oz.)	43	1	9	24	258	0.52
Caviar, black and red, granular (1 oz.)	530	0	78	85	101	0.27
Clam, mixed species, canned, drained solids (3 oz.)	485	19	78	15	287	2.32
Clam, mixed species, breaded and fried (3 oz.)	257	9	54	12	160	1.24
Cod, Atlantic, cooked, dry heat (1 fillet)	83	2	25	76	248	1.04
Cod liver oil (1 tbsp.)	13,600	0	0	0	0	0
Crab						
Alaska king, cooked, moist heat (3 oz.)	25	7	50	54	238	6.48
Alaska king, imitation, made from surimi (3 oz.)	56	0	11	37	240	0.28
Baked (1 crab)	77	3	415	82	337	7.02
Cake (1 cake)	313	0	202	25	227	2.12
Blue, canned (3 oz.)	4	2	86	33	221	3.42
Dungeness, cooked, moist heat (1 crab)	132	5	75	74	222	6.95
Soft-shell, fried (1 crab)	15	1	55	25	131	1.06

	VIT A (IU)	VIT C (mg)	CAL (mg)	MAG (mg)	PHOS (mg)	ZINC (mg)
Crayfish, mixed species, farmed, cooked, moist heat (3 oz.)	43	0	43	28	205	1.26
Cod, Pacific, cooked, dry heat (3 oz.)	27	3	8	26	190	0.43
Dolphinfish, cooked, dry heat (3 oz.)	177	0	16	32	156	0.5
Fish fillet, battered or breaded, and fried (1 fillet)	35	0	16	22	156	0.4
Fish sticks, breaded, frozen (1 oz.)	30	*	6	7	51	0.19
Grouper, mixed species, cooked, dry heat (1 fillet)	333	0	42	75	289	1.03
Halibut, Greenland, cooked, dry heat (3 oz.)	51	0	3	28	179	0.43
Lobster, Northern, cooked, moist heat (3 oz.)	74	0	52	30	157	2.48
Lobster, spiny, mixed species, cooked, moist heat (3 oz.)	17	2	54	43	195	6.18
Herring, Atlantic, cooked, dry heat (3 oz.)	87	1	63	35	258	1.08
Herring, Atlantic, kippered (1 oz.)	36	0	24	13	92	0.39
Herring, Pacific, cooked, dry heat (3 oz.)	99	0	90	35	248	0.58
Mackerel, king, cooked, dry heat (3 oz.)	713	1	34	35	270	0.61
Monkfish, cooked, dry heat (3 oz.)	39	1	9	23	218	0.45

	VIT A (IU)	VIT C (mg)	CAL (mg)	MAG (mg)	PHOS (mg)	ZINC (mg)
Ocean perch, Atlantic, cooked, dry heat (3 oz.)	39	1	117	33	236	0.52
Oyster, Eastern, canned (3 oz.)	255	4	38	46	118	77.31
Perch, mixed species, cooked, dry heat (3 oz.)	27	2	87	32	219	1.22
Pompano, Florida, cooked, dry heat (1 fillet)	106	0	38	27	300	0.61
Red snapper, cooked, dry heat (3 oz.)	326	1	34	31	*	*
Rockfish, cooked, dry heat (3 oz.)	326	1	10	29	*	*
Roe, mixed species, cooked, dry heat (3 oz.)	258	14	24	22	438	1.09
Roughy, orange, cooked, dry heat (3 oz.)	69	0	32	32	218	0.82
Roughy, orange, raw (3 oz.)	60	0	26	26	170	0.64
Salmon, Atlantic, farmed, cooked, dry heat (3 oz.)	43	3	13	26	214	0.37
Salmon, Atlantic, wild, cooked, dry heat (3 oz.)	37	0	13	32	218	0.7
Salmon, chinook, cooked, dry heat (3 oz.)	422	4	24	104	315	0.48
Salmon, chinook, smoked (3 oz.)	75	0	9	15	139	0.26
Salmon, chum, drained solids with bone and liquid (3 oz.)	52	0	212	26	301	0.85

	VIT A (IU)	VIT C (mg)	CAL (mg)	MAG (mg)	PHOS (mg)	ZINC (mg)
Salmon, pink, canned, solids with bone and liquid (3 oz.)	47	0	181	29	280	0.78
Salmon, pink, cooked, dry heat (3 oz.)	116	0	15	28	251	0.6
Sardines, Atlantic, canned in oil, drained solids with bone (3.75 oz.)	206	0	351	36	451	1.21
Sardines, fish oil (1 tbsp.)	0	0	0	0	0	0
Sardines, Pacific, canned in tomato sauce, drained solids with bone (1 cup)	325	1	214	30	326	1.25
Scallop, mixed species, breaded and fried (2 large scallops)	23	1	13	18	73	0.33
Sea bass, mixed species, cooked, dry heat (3 oz.)	181	0	11	45	211	0.44
Sea trout, mixed species, cooked, dry heat (3 oz.)	98	0	19	34	273	0.49
Sea trout, mixed species, raw (3 oz.)	85	0	15	26	213	0.38
Shad, American, cooked, dry heat (3 oz.)	102	0	51	32	297	0.4
Shark fin, prepared (1 cup)	0	0	22	15	45	1.77
Shark, mixed species, battered-dipped and fried (3 oz.)	153	0	43	37	165	0.41
Shark, mixed species, raw (100 g)	233	0	34	49	210	0.43

	VIT A (IU)	VIT C (mg)	CAL (mg)	MAG (mg)	PHOS (mg)	ZINC (mg)
Shrimp, mixed species, canned (3 oz.)	51	2	50	35	198	1.07
Shrimp, mixed species, breaded and fried (3 oz.)	161	1	57	34	185	1.17
Shrimp, mixed species, cooked, moist heat (3 oz.)	186	2	33	29	117	1.33
Snapper, mixed species, cooked, dry heat (3 oz.)	98	1	34	32	171	0.37
Sturgeon, cooked, dry heat (3 oz.)	*	*	11	30	*	*
Surimi, imitation crab and lobster (3 oz.)	57	*	8	37	*	*
Sunfish, pumpkin-seed, cooked, dry heat (3 oz.)	49	1	88	32	196	1.69
Swordfish, cooked, dry heat (3 oz.)	117	1	5	29	287	1.25
Trout, mixed species, cooked, dry heat (3 oz.)	54	0	47	24	267	0.72
Trout, rainbow, farmed, cooked, dry heat (3 oz.)	244	3	73	27	226	0.42
Tuna, light, canned in oil, drained, solids (3 oz.)	66	0	11	26	264	0.77
Tuna, light, canned in water, drained, solids (3 oz.)	48	0	9	23	139	0.66
Tuna, white, canned in oil, drained, solids (3 oz.)	68	0	3	29	227	0.4
Tuna, white, canned in water, drained solids (3 oz.)	16	0	12	28	185	0.41

	VIT A (IU)	VIT C (mg)	CAL (mg)	MAG (mg)	PHOS (mg)	ZINC (mg)
Tuna, yellowfin, fresh, cooked, dry heat (3 oz.)	58	1	18	54	208	0.57
Turbot, European, cooked, dry heat (3 oz.)	34	2	20	55	140	0.24
Yellowtail, mixed species, cooked, dry heat (3 oz.)	88	3	25	32	171	0.57
White perch, filet, fried (3 oz.)	8	*	12	*	*	*
Whitefish, mixed species, cooked, dry heat (3 oz.)	111	0	28	36	294	1.08
Whitefish, mixed species, smoked (3 oz.)	162	0	15	20	112	0.42
Vegetarian, tuna, Worthington (½ cup)	0	0	20	*	88	0.4

SNACK FOODS

	VIT A (IU)	VIT C (mg)	CAL (mg)	MAG (mg)	PHOS (mg)	ZINC (mg)
Banana chips (3 oz.)	71	5	15	65	48	0.64
Beef jerky, chopped and formed (1 oz.)	0	0	6	15	115	2.3
Chex mix (1 oz., approx. ⅔ cup)	41	14	10	18	53	0.59
Combos, Cheddar Cheese Pretzel (10 Combos)	20	0	59	7	43	0.22
Corn chips, barbecue-flavor (7 oz.)	1210	3	259	153	410	2.1
Corn chips, plain (7 oz.)	186	0	252	151	366	2.5
Corn puffs, cheese-flavor (1 oz.)	75	0	16	5	31	0.11

	VIT A (IU)	VIT C (mg)	CAL (mg)	MAG (mg)	PHOS (mg)	ZINC (mg)
Corn twists, cheese-flavor (1 cup)	602	1	132	41	245	0.86
Cornnuts						
Barbecue-flavor (1 oz.)	96	0	5	31	80	0.53
Nacho-flavor (1 oz.)	11	4	10	31	88	0.51
Plain (1 oz.)	0	0	3	32	78	0.51
Doo Dads snack mix, original flavor (½ cup)	43	0	21	17	84	0.64
Doughnuts, cake-type, plain, glazed or sugared (1 medium doughnut)	5	0	27	8	53	0.2
Ice cream cones, cake, wafer-type (1 cone)	0	0	1	1	4	0.03
Ice cream cones, sugar, rolled-type (1 cone)	0	0	4	3	10	0.08
Oriental mix, rice-based (1 oz.)	1	0	15	34	74	0.75
Sesame sticks, wheat-based, salted (1 oz.)	25	0	48	13	39	0.33
Sweet Potato Chips, Terra Chips, Dana Alexander, Inc. (1 oz.)	4000	0	20	*	*	*
Tortilla chips, nacho flavor (1 cup)	842	4	334	186	554	2.72
Tortilla chips, plain (7½ oz. bag)	418	0	328	187	437	3.26
Trail mix, regular (1 cup)	27	2	117	237	518	4.83
Trail mix, regular, with chocolate chips, salted nuts, and seeds (1 oz.)	13	0	31	46	110	0.89
Trail mix, tropical (1 oz.)	14	2	16	27	53	0.33

	VIT A (IU)	VIT C (mg)	CAL (mg)	MAG (mg)	PHOS (mg)	ZINC (mg)
Tortilla chips, plain (1 oz.)	56	0	44	25	58	0.43

Frozen snacks *(see also* Desserts)

	VIT A (IU)	VIT C (mg)	CAL (mg)	MAG (mg)	PHOS (mg)	ZINC (mg)
Fruit Juice bars, grape, frozen, (1 bar)	0	18	0	0	0	0
Fruit leather bars, with cream (1 bar)	13	15	5	3	7	0.04
Ice Cream						
Chocolate (½ cup)	275	1	72	19	71	0.38
Chocolate, low-fat (½ cup)	270	*	85	9	69	0.45
Vanilla (½ cup)	270	0	85	9	69	0.46
Ice milk, vanilla, soft-serve (½ cup)	91	1	138	12	107	0.05
Italian ice, (½ cup)	194	1	1	0	0	0.04
Sherbet, lemon (½ cup)	87	8	40	*	*	*
Sorbet, orange (1 cup)	70	6	60	*	*	*
Yogurt, vanilla, soft-serve (½ cup)	153	1	103	10	93	0.03

Granola Bars

	VIT A (IU)	VIT C (mg)	CAL (mg)	MAG (mg)	PHOS (mg)	ZINC (mg)
Crunchy Almond/Brown Sugar, Low-fat, Kellogg (1 bar)	2381	0	35	87	248	2.2
Hard, chocolate chip (1 bar)	10	0	18	17	48	0.46
Hard, plain (1 bar, 1 oz.)	43	0	17	28	79	0.58
Nutri-Grain Cereal Bars, fruit, Kellogg (100 g)	2027	0	41	27	103	4.1
Soft, milk chocolate coating, chocolate chip (1 bar, 1.25 oz.)	14	0	37	23	70	0.46
Soft, milk chocolate coating, peanut butter (1 bar)	48	0	40	25	83	0.54

	VIT A (IU)	VIT C (mg)	CAL (mg)	MAG (mg)	PHOS (mg)	ZINC (mg)
Soft, uncoated, nut and raisin (1 bar, 1 oz.)	12	0	24	26	68	0.45
Soft, uncoated, peanut butter (1 bar, 1 oz.)	4	0	26	24	71	0.53
Soft, uncoated, raisin (1 bar, 1.5 oz.)	0	0	43	31	94	0.55
Popcorn						
Air-popped (1 cup)	16	0	1	11	24	0.28
Air-popped, white popcorn (1 cup)	2	0	1	11	24	0.28
Cakes (1 cake)	7	0	1	16	28	0.4
Caramel-coated, with peanuts (1 oz., 2/3 cup)	18	0	19	23	36	0.35
Caramel-coated, without peanuts (1 oz.)	14	0	12	10	24	0.16
Cheese-flavor (1 cup)	27	0	12	10	40	0.22
Oil-popped (1 cup)	17	0	1	12	28	0.29
White cheddar (1 cup)	114	2	28	21	*	*
Potato chips						
Made from dried potatoes, cheese flavor (1 oz.)	0	2	31	15	46	0.18
Made from dried potatoes, light (1 oz.)	0	3	10	18	44	0.17
Made from dried potatoes, plain (1 oz.)	0	2	7	16	45	0.17
Made from dried potatoes, sour cream and onion flavor (1 oz.)	214	3	18	16	48	0.2

	VIT A (IU)	VIT C (mg)	CAL (mg)	MAG (mg)	PHOS (mg)	ZINC (mg)
Plain, light (1 oz.)	0	6	10	18	*	*
Plain, made with partially hydrogenated soybean oil, salted (1 cup)	0	71	54	152	375	2.47
Plain, unsalted (1 cup)	0	71	55	152	375	2.47
Potato sticks (1 oz.)	0	13	5	18	49	0.28

Pretzels

	VIT A (IU)	VIT C (mg)	CAL (mg)	MAG (mg)	PHOS (mg)	ZINC (mg)
Hard, plain, made with enriched flour, salted (1 oz.)	0	0	10	10	32	0.24
Hard, plain, salted (1 oz.)	0	0	10	10	32	0.24
Hard, plain, salted (10 twists)	0	0	22	21	68	0.51
Hard, whole wheat (1 oz.)	0	0	8	9	35	0.18
Rice bar, crisped, chocolate chip (1 bar, 1 oz.)	500	0	6	14	38	0.24
Rice cakes, brown rice, multigrain, unsalted (1 cake)	0	0	2	12	33	0.23
Rice cakes, brown rice, plain (1 cake)	4	0	1	12	32	0.27
Rice Krispies Treats Squares, Kellogg's (100 g)	909	0	3	13	42	0.5

Snack bars *(see also* Granola bars)

	VIT A (IU)	VIT C (mg)	CAL (mg)	MAG (mg)	PHOS (mg)	ZINC (mg)
Chocolate (1 bar)	1166	21	29	19	*	*
Chocolate chip (1 bar)	1166	21	29	19	*	*
Chocolate chip crunch (1 bar)	500	9	150	24	*	*

	VIT A (IU)	VIT C (mg)	CAL (mg)	MAG (mg)	PHOS (mg)	ZINC (mg)
Fat-free (1 bar)	333	*	20	*	*	*
Honey oats (1 bar)	833	*	0	24	*	8
Nutri-Grain (1 bar)	500	*	16	10	*	*
Peanut butter crunch (1 bar)	500	9	150	24	*	*
Vanilla crunch (1 bar)	500	9	150	24	*	*
Yogurt (1 bar)	67	9	60	*	*	*

SOUPS

	VIT A (IU)	VIT C (mg)	CAL (mg)	MAG (mg)	PHOS (mg)	ZINC (mg)
Bean with bacon (1 cup)	889	2	81	44	132	1.03
Beef bouillon, powder, dry (1 cube)	2	0	2	2	12	0
Beef broth, powder, dry (1 cube)	2	0	2	2	12	0
Beef noodle, (1 cup)	629	0	15	6	46	1.54
Black bean canned, condensed, commercial (1 cup)	1144	1	90	85	193	2.83
Black turtle soup, mature seeds, canned (1 cup)	10	7	84	84	259	1.3
Cheese, canned, condensed, commercial (1 cup)	2177	0	285	8	272	1.29
Chicken noodle, canned, condensed, commercial (1 cup)	1309	0	27	10	74	0.57
Chicken rice, canned, chunky, ready-to-serve (1 cup)	5858	4	34	10	72	0.96
Chicken Rice with Vegetables, canned, ready-to-serve, Progresso Healthy Classics (100 g)	688	0	10	10	37	0.18

	VIT A (IU)	VIT C (mg)	CAL (mg)	MAG (mg)	PHOS (mg)	ZINC (mg)
Chicken vegetable, canned, chunky, ready-to-serve (1 cup)	5990	6	26	10	106	2.16
Chicken with dumplings, canned, condensed, commercial (1 cup)	1041	0	30	7	123	0.74
Chili beef, canned, condensed (1 cup)	3022	8	87	61	297	2.8
Clam chowder, Manhattan style, canned, chunky, ready-to-serve (1 cup)	3293	12	67	19	84	1.68
Clam chowder, New England, canned, condensed, commercial (1 cup)	20	5	82	15	85	1.51
Clam chowder, New England, made with milk (1 cup)	164	4	187	23	157	0.8
Consommé with gelatin, dehydrated, prepared (1 cup)	8	0	8	8	40	0
Corn chowder (1 cup)	450	39	73	31	*	*
Crab, ready to serve (1 cup)	170	*	66	88	*	*
Cream of asparagus, canned, condensed, commercial (1 cup)	891	6	58	8	78	1.76
Cream of asparagus, canned, prepared with equal volume milk, commercial (1 cup)	600	4	174	20	154	0.93

	VIT A (IU)	VIT C (mg)	CAL (mg)	MAG (mg)	PHOS (mg)	ZINC (mg)
Cream of broccoli, canned, ready-to-serve, Progresso Healthy Classics (100 g)	120	2	17	6	16	0.11
Cream of broccoli, Campbell's Restaurant Soup (½ cup)	0	12	80	*	*	*
Cream of celery, canned, condensed, commercial (1 cup)	612	1	80	13	75	0.3
Cream of celery, canned, prepared with equal volume milk, commercial (1 cup)	461	1	186	22	151	0.2
Cream of chicken, canned, condensed, commercial (1 cup)	1123	0	68	5	75	1.26
Cream of chicken, prepared with equal volume milk, commercial (1 cup)	714	1	181	17	151	0.68
Cream of mushroom, canned, condensed, commercial (1 cup)	0	2	65	10	85	1.19
Cream of mushroom, canned, prepared with equal volume milk commercial (1 cup)	154	2	179	20	156	0.64
Cream of potato, canned, condensed (1 cup)	577	0	40	3	93	1.26

	VIT A (IU)	VIT C (mg)	CAL (mg)	MAG (mg)	PHOS (mg)	ZINC (mg)
Cream of potato, canned, prepared with equal volume milk, commercial (1 cup)	444	1	166	17	161	0.68
Cream of shrimp, canned, prepared with equal volume milk, commercial (1 cup)	313	1	164	22	146	0.8
Cream of vegetable, dehydrated, dry (1 packet)	27	3	24	9	40	0.28
Escarole, canned, ready-to-serve (1 cup)	2170	5	32	5	79	2.23
Gazpacho, canned, ready-to-serve (1 cup)	2604	7	24	7	37	0.24
Garlic and Pasta, canned, ready-to-serve, Progresso Healthy Classics (100 g)	1270	0	21	14	36	0.23
Lentil with ham, canned, ready-to-serve (1 cup)	360	4	42	22	184	0.74
Minestrone, canned, chunky, ready-to-serve (1 cup)	4351	5	60	14	110	1.44
Mushroom, dehydrated, dry (1 instant packet)	5	1	51	4	59	0.07
Mushroom, dehydrated, dry (1 regular packet)	22	4	228	18	263	0.3
Onion mix, dehydrated, dry (1 packet)	8	1	55	25	126	0.23

	VIT A (IU)	VIT C (mg)	CAL (mg)	MAG (mg)	PHOS (mg)	ZINC (mg)
Oyster stew, made with water	71	3	22	5	48	10.29
Oyster stew, made with milk (1 cup)	225	4	167	21	162	10.34
Pea, green, canned, prepared with equal volume milk, commercial (1 cup)	356	3	173	56	239	1.76
Pea, split, with ham, canned, chunky ready-to-serve (1 cup)	4872	7	34	38	178	3.12
Pepper pot (1 cup)	865	1	23	5	42	1.22
Tomato, canned, prepared with equal volume milk, commercial (1 cup)	848	68	159	22	149	0.29
Tomato and rice (1 cup)	755	0	23	5	33	0.51
Tomato beef with noodle (1 cup)	533	0	18	8	56	0.75
Tomato bisque, prepared with water (1 cup)	721	6	40	9	60	0.59
Tomato bisque, prepared with milk (1 cup)	879	7	186	25	174	0.63
Tomato bisque, with rice (1 cup)	755	15	23	5	33	0.51
Tomato bisque, with whole milk, (1 cup)	879	15	186	25	174	0.63
Tomato vegetable, prepared (1 cup)	850	5	8	20	*	*
Turkey noodle, canned, condensed commercial (1 cup)	585	0	23	10	95	1.17
Turkey, chunky (1 cup)	7156	6	50	na	104	2.12

	VIT A (IU)	VIT C (mg)	CAL (mg)	MAG (mg)	PHOS (mg)	ZINC (mg)
Vegetable with beef broth, canned condensed, commercial (1 cup)	4199	5	34	12	79	1.6
Vegetarian vegetable, canned, condensed, commercial (1 cup)	6034	3	42	15	69	0.92

SOY

	VIT A (IU)	VIT C (mg)	CAL (mg)	MAG (mg)	PHOS (mg)	ZINC (mg)
Fuyu, tofu, salted and fermented, prepared with calcium sulfate (1 block)	18	0	135	6	8	0.17
Koyadofu, tofu, dried-frozen (1 piece, 17 g)	88	0	62	10	82	0.83
Koyadofu, tofu, dried-frozen, prepared with calcium sulfate (1 piece, 17 g)	88	0	363	31	82	0.83
Miso, fermented soybeans (1 cup)	239	0	182	116	421	9.13
Natto, soybean product (1 cup)	0	23	380	201	305	5.3
Soybean, oil, salad or cooking (1 tbsp.)	0	0	0	0	0	0
Okara, tofu (1 cup)	0	0	98	32	73	0.68

Soybeans (see Soy for additional items)

	VIT A (IU)	VIT C (mg)	CAL (mg)	MAG (mg)	PHOS (mg)	ZINC (mg)
Boiled (½ cup)	8	6	88	74	211	0.99
Boiled (1 cup)	16	12	176	148	422	1.98
Dried, uncooked (½ cup)	22	6	257	261	654	4.54
Dried, uncooked (1 cup)	44	12	514	522	1,308	9.08
Green, boiled, drained, without salt (1 cup)	281	31	261	108	284	1.64

	VIT A (IU)	VIT C (mg)	CAL (mg)	MAG (mg)	PHOS (mg)	ZINC (mg)
Green, fresh, boiled, drained (½ cup)	140	15	130	*	142	*
Green, fresh, raw (½ cup)	230	37	252	*	248	*
Green, raw (1 cup)	461	74	504	166	497	2.53
Mature seeds, boiled, with salt (1 cup)	16	3	175	148	421	1.98
Mature seeds, dry, roasted (1 cup)	40	8	464	392	1116	8.2
Mature seeds, roasted, salted (1 cup)	344	4	237	249	624	5.4
Mature seeds, sprouted, steamed (1 cup)	10	8	56	56	127	0.98
Mature seeds, sprouted, stir-fried (100 g)	17	12	82	96	216	2.1
Mature seeds, sprouted, raw (½ cup)	4	5	24	25	57	0.41
Organically produced, Arrowhead Mills, unprepared (¼ cup)	0	0	100	*	*	*
Roasted (½ cup)	172	2	119	125	312	2.7
Soybean cakes						
Chinese style, extra firm (3 oz.)	0	0	150	*	*	*
Japanese style, firm (3 oz.)	0	0	150	*	*	*
Kinugoshi, silken (3 oz.)	0	0	20	*	*	*
Sprouted, raw (½ cup)	4	5	23	25	57	0.41
Sprouted, steamed (½ cup)	5	4	28	28	63	0.49

Soy Beverages

	VIT A (IU)	VIT C (mg)	CAL (mg)	MAG (mg)	PHOS (mg)	ZINC (mg)
Edensoy Organic Soy Beverage						
Carob, (1 cup)	*	*	68	43	105	0.64
Original (1 cup)	*	*	82	55	143	0.98

	VIT A (IU)	VIT C (mg)	CAL (mg)	MAG (mg)	PHOS (mg)	ZINC (mg)
Original, Extra (1 cup)	1176	*	196	54	142	1
Vanilla (1 cup)	*	*	62	38	98	0.58
Vanilla Extra (1 cup)	1176	*	196	38	294	0.57
Soy milk (1 cup)	77	*	10	45	117	0.54
Soy Moo, Fat-free, nondairy, lactose-free (1 cup)	0	0	400	*	*	*
Soy protein isolate (1 oz.)	0	0	50	11	220	1.14
Soy Protein Isolate Powder, Vitamin World, Isoflavones and Geristein, unprepared (1 scoop)	0	0	60	60	200	*
Tempeh (½ cup)	569	0	77	58	171	1.5
Tempeh, soybean product (1 cup)	1139	0	154	116	342	3.01
Tofu						
Fried, prepared with calcium sulfate (1 piece)	0	0	125	12	37	0.26
Koyadofu, dried-frozen (1 piece)	88	0	363	31	82	0.83
Koyadofu, dried-frozen (¼ lb)	587	1	412	67	545	5.5
Raw, firm (½ cup)	209	0	258	118	239	1.98
Raw, firm, prepared with calcium sulfate (½ cup)	209	0	861	73	239	1.98
Raw, regular (1 cup)	211	0	260	255	241	1.98
Raw, regular, prepared with calcium sulfate (½ cup)	105	0	434	37	120	0.99
Regular (½ cup)	105	0	130	127	120	1

	VIT A (IU)	VIT C (mg)	CAL (mg)	MAG (mg)	PHOS (mg)	ZINC (mg)
Silken (3 oz.)	0	0	20	*	*	*
Silken, Lite, Low-Fat, Firm, Mori-Nu (3 oz.)	0	0	20	*	*	*

VEGETABLES, FRESH

	VIT A (IU)	VIT C (mg)	CAL (mg)	MAG (mg)	PHOS (mg)	ZINC (mg)
Alfalfa seeds, fresh, sprouted (1 cup)	50	3	10	9	23	0.3
Artichoke, boiled (1 med.)	212	12	54	72	103	0.59
Artichoke hearts (1/2 cup)	149	8	38	51	72	0.44
Arugula, raw (1/2 cup)	237	2	16	5	5	0.05
Asparagus, boiled, drained (1/2 cup)	485	10	18	9	49	0.38
Balsam-pear, pods, boiled, drained (1/2 cup)	70	21	5	10	22	0.43
Balsam-pear, pods, boiled, drained (1 cup)	140	41	11	20	45	0.95
Bamboo shoots, boiled (1/2 cup)	0	0	7	2	12	*
Beans						
Adzuki, mature seeds, boiled (1 cup)	14	0	64	120	386	4.07
Baked, home-prepared (1 cup)	0	3	154	109	276	1.85
Black, mature seeds, boiled (1 cup)	10	0	46	120	241	1.93
Broad, immature seeds, boiled, drained (100 g)	270	20	18	31	73	0.47

	VIT A (IU)	VIT C (mg)	CAL (mg)	MAG (mg)	PHOS (mg)	ZINC (mg)
Chickpeas, (garbanzo beans bengal gram), mature seeds, boiled (1 cup)	44	2	80	79	276	2.51
Cranberry, (Roman), mature seeds, boiled (1 cup)	0	0	89	89	239	2.02
French, mature seeds, boiled (1 cup)	5	2	112	99	181	1.13
Great Northern, mature seeds, boiled (1 cup)	2	2	120	89	292	1.56
Kidney, California red, mature seeds, boiled (1 cup)	5	2	117	85	242	1.52
Kidney, all types, mature seeds, boiled (1 cup)	0	2	50	80	251	1.89
Limas						
Baby, frozen (½ cup)	150	5	25	50	101	0.5
Dried, boiled (½ cup)	0	0	16	41	104	0.89
Fresh (½ cup)	315	9	27	63	111	0.67
Fordhook, frozen (½ cup)	160	11	19	29	54	0.37
Mung, dehydrated (1 cup)	0	0	35	4	45	0.57
Mung, mature seeds, sprouted, raw (1 cup)	22	14	14	22	56	0.43
Navy, mature seeds, boiled (1 cup)	4	2	127	107	286	1.93
Pink, mature seeds, boiled (1 cup)	0	0	88	110	279	1.62

	VIT A (IU)	VIT C (mg)	CAL (mg)	MAG (mg)	PHOS (mg)	ZINC (mg)
Pinto, immature seeds, frozen, boiled, drained (1/3 of 10 oz. package)	0	1	49	51	94	0.65
Pinto, mature seeds, boiled (1 cup)	3	4	82	94	274	1.85
Snap, green, boiled, drained (1 cup)	833	12	58	31	49	0.45
Snap, green, fresh, boiled (1/2 cup)	413	6	29	16	24	0.23
Snap, yellow, boiled, (1 cup)	101	12	58	31	49	0.45
Small white, mature seeds, cooked (1 cup)	0	0	131	122	303	1.95
Yam beans, fresh, raw, trimmed, sliced (1 cup)	25	24	14	14	21	0.19
Yard-long, fresh, boiled, drained, sliced (1/2 cup)	234	8	23	22	30	*
Yard-long, dried, boiled (1/2 cup)	14	*	36	84	156	0.92
Yellow, dried, boiled (1/2 cup)	2	2	66	61	152	0.98
White, regular, dried, boiled (1/2 cup)	0	0	81	57	102	1.24
White, small, boiled (1/2 cup)	0	0	66	61	152	0.98
Winged, boiled, drained (1/2 cup)	27	3	19	9	8	*
Winged, dried, boiled (1/2 cup)	0	0	122	47	132	1.24
Beet greens, raw (1 cup)	2318	11	45	27	15	0.14
Beets, boiled, drained (1/2 cup)	30	3	14	20	32	0.3

	VIT A (IU)	VIT C (mg)	CAL (mg)	MAG (mg)	PHOS (mg)	ZINC (mg)
Bok choy, Chinese cabbage, cooked (1 cup)	5050	26	250	*	*	*
Broccoli						
Flowerets, raw (1 cup)	1095	66	34	18	47	0.28
Frozen, spears, boiled, drained (1/2 cup)	1741	37	47	18	51	0.28
Frozen, chopped, boiled, drained (1 cup)	3481	74	94	37	101	0.55
Brussels sprouts, frozen, boiled, drained (1 cup)	913	71	37	37	84	0.56
Cabbage						
Boiled, drained (1/2 cup)	99	15	23	6	11	0.07
Chinese (pak-choi), boiled (1 cup)	4366	44	158	19	49	0.29
Chinese (pak-choi), raw (1 cup)	2100	32	74	13	26	0.13
Chinese (pe-tsai), boiled, drained, shredded (1 cup)	1151	19	38	12	46	0.21
Chinese (pe-tsai), raw, shredded (1 cup)	912	21	59	10	22	0.18
Marinated, Kim Chee (1/2 cup)	750	6	*	*	*	*
Raw (1 cup)	93	23	33	11	16	0.13
Red, boiled, drained, shredded (1/2 cup)	20	26	28	8	22	0.11
Red, raw, shredded (1 cup)	28	40	36	11	29	0.15
Savoy, raw, shredded (1 cup)	700	22	25	20	29	0.19

	VIT A (IU)	VIT C (mg)	CAL (mg)	MAG (mg)	PHOS (mg)	ZINC (mg)
Swamp cabbage, (skunk cabbage) raw, chopped (1 cup)	3528	31	43	40	22	0.1
Cactus, tender strips (2 tsp.)	100	*	*	*	*	*
Carrots						
Boiled, drained (1/2 cup, slices)	19,152	2	24	10	23	0.23
Raw (1 medium)	17,159	6	16	9	27	0.12
Raw, baby (1 medium)	197	1	2	1	4	0.02
Shredded (1 cup)	10,303	10	30	17	*	*
Cassava, raw (1 cup)	21	99	188	136	144	0.52
Cauliflower						
Frozen, boiled, drained (1 cup, 1" pieces)	40	56	31	16	43	0.23
Green, cooked (1/5 head)	127	65	29	17	51	0.57
Green, raw (1 cup)	97	56	21	13	40	0.41
Raw (1 cup)	19	46	22	15	44	0.28
Celeriac, raw (1 cup)	0	13	67	31	179	0.52
Celery, raw (1 cup, diced)	161	8	48	13	30	0.16
Chicory greens, raw, chopped (1 cup)	7200	43	180	54	85	0.76
Chicory roots, raw (1/2 cup, 1" pieces)	3	2	18	10	27	0.15
Chives, raw, chopped (1 tbsp.)	131	2	3	1	2	0.02
Collards, chopped, boiled, drained (100 g, or about 5/8 cup)	598	26	210	30	27	0.27

	VIT A (IU)	VIT C (mg)	CAL (mg)	MAG (mg)	PHOS (mg)	ZINC (mg)
Corn						
Yellow, sweet, boiled, drained (½ cup cut)	178	5	2	26	84	0.39
Yellow, sweet, raw (1 medium ear)	253	6	2	33	80	0.41
White, frozen, kernels cut off cob, boiled (½ cup)	0	3	3	16	47	0.33
Cowpeas, common, (black-eyed crowder, Southern), mature seeds, boiled (1 cup)	26	1	41	91	268	2.22
Cowpeas, cooked, chopped (1 cup)	305	10	37	33	22	0.13
Cress, garden, raw (1 cup)	4650	35	41	19	38	0.12
Cucumber, with peel, raw, slices (½ cup)	112	3	7	6	10	0.1
Dandelion greens, raw, chopped (1 cup)	7700	19	103	20	36	0.23
Eggplant, boiled, drained, cubes (1 cup)	63	1	6	13	22	0.15
Endive, raw, chopped (½ cup)	513	2	13	4	7	0.2
Fennel, bulb, raw, sliced (1 cup)	117	10	43	15	44	0.17
Gingeroot, raw, sliced (¼ cup)	0	1	4	10	7	*
Horseradish, leafy tips, boiled, drained, chopped (1 cup)	2946	13	63	63	28	0.21
Horseradish-tree, pods, raw, slices (1 cup)	74	141	30	45	50	0.45
Hummus, garbanzo (½ cup)	31	10	62	36	138	1.35

	VIT A (IU)	VIT C (mg)	CAL (mg)	MAG (mg)	PHOS (mg)	ZINC (mg)
Hummus, garbanzo (1 cup)	61	19	124	71	275	2.7
Jerusalem artichoke, raw, slices (1 cup)	30	6	21	26	117	0.18
Jicama, raw (1 cup)	25	43	17	13	32	*
Kale, boiled, drained chopped (1 cup)	9620	53	94	23	36	0.31
Kale, frozen, boiled, drained, chopped (1 cup)	8260	33	179	23	36	0.23
Kohlrabi, boiled (1 cup)	29	44	20	16	39	*
Kohlrabi, raw (1/2 cup)	25	43	17	13	32	*
Leeks (bulb and lower leaf portion), drained, chopped, or diced, boiled (1/4 cup)	12	1	8	4	4	0.02
Leeks (bulb and lower leaf portion), raw (1 cup)	85	11	53	25	31	0.11
Lentils, mature seeds, boiled (1/2 cup)	8	2	18	36	122	1.26
Lentils, mature seeds, boiled (1 cup)	16	3	38	71	356	2.52
Lentils, sprouted, raw (1 cup)	35	13	19	29	133	1.16
Lettuce						
Butterhead (includes Boston and bibb types), raw, shredded (1 cup)	534	4	18	7	13	0.09
Cos, or romaine, raw, shredded (1/2 cup)	728	7	10	2	13	0.07
Iceberg, includes crisphead types raw, shredded (1 cup)	182	2	11	5	11	0.12

	VIT A (IU)	VIT C (mg)	CAL (mg)	MAG (mg)	PHOS (mg)	ZINC (mg)
Looseleaf, raw, shredded (½ cup)	532	5	19	3	7	0.08
Lotus root, raw (10 slices)	0	36	36	19	81	0.32
Mushroom						
Enoki, raw (1 large)	0	1	0	1	6	0.03
Raw, pieces or slices, (1 cup)	0	3	4	7	73	0.51
Shiitake, dried (4 mushrooms)	0	1	2	20	44	1.15
White, raw, chopped (1 cup)	0	2	1	*	*	*
Mustard greens, boiled, drained, chopped (1 cup)	4243	35	104	21	57	0.15
Mustard greens, frozen, cooked, drained, chopped (1 cup)	6705	21	152	20	36	0.3
Mustard spinach, tendergreen, boiled, drained, chopped (1 cup)	14,760	117	284	13	32	0.2
Nopales, cooked (1 cup)	684	8	244	70	24	0.31
Okra, raw, sliced (1 cup)	660	*	81	57	63	0.6
Onions, dehydrated flakes (¼ cup)	0	11	36	13	42	0.27
Onions, raw (1 large slice, ¼″ thick)	0	2	8	3	13	0.07
Parsley, freeze-dried (¼ cup)	885	2	3	5	8	0.09
Parsley, raw (1 cup)	3120	80	82	30	35	0.64
Parsnips, raw, slices (1 cup)	0	23	48	39	94	0.79
Peas						
Cooked, podded (1 cup)	210	77	67	42	88	0.59

	VIT A (IU)	VIT C (mg)	CAL (mg)	MAG (mg)	PHOS (mg)	ZINC (mg)
Green, boiled, drained (1 cup)	955	23	43	62	187	1.9
Green, frozen, boiled, drained (1/2 cup)	534	8	19	23	72	0.75
Split, dried, boiled (1/2 cup)	7	*	13	36	97	0.98
Split, mature seeds, boiled (1 cup)	14	1	27	71	194	1.96
Sprouted, mature seeds, raw (1/2 cup)	100	6	21	34	99	0.63
Peas and carrots, frozen, boiled, drained (1/2 cup)	6209	7	18	13	39	0.36
Peas and onions, frozen, boiled, drained (1 cup)	625	12	25	23	61	0.52
Peppers						
Hot chili, green, raw (1 pepper)	347	109	8	11	21	0.14
Hot chili, red, raw (1 pepper)	4838	109	8	11	21	0.14
Hot chili, sun-dried (1 pepper)	143	0	0	1	1	0.01
Sweet, red, raw (1 medium)	6783	226	11	12	23	0.14
Sweet, green, raw (1 medium)	752	106	11	12	23	0.14
Sweet, yellow, raw (1 large pepper)	443	341	21	22	45	0.32
Pickle, cucumber, dill (1 large)	214	1	6	7	14	0.09
Pickle, cucumber, sweet (1 large)	44	0	1	1	4	0.03
Pigeon peas, mature seeds, cooked, boiled (1 cup)	5	0	72	77	200	1.51

	VIT A (IU)	VIT C (mg)	CAL (mg)	MAG (mg)	PHOS (mg)	ZINC (mg)
Poi, taro root (1 cup)	16	10	37	58	*	*
Potatoes						
Boiled, cooked in skin, flesh (1 potato, 2½″ dia.)	0	18	7	30	60	0.41
Boiled, cooked without skin (1 potato, 2½″ dia.)	0	10	11	27	54	0.37
Raw, flesh and skin (1 large)	0	36	13	39	85	0.72
Pumpkin, boiled, drained, mashed (½ cup)	1320	6	18	11	37	*
Pumpkin, raw (1 cup, 1″ cubes)	1856	10	24	14	51	0.37
Radicchio, raw, shredded (1 cup)	11	3	8	5	16	0.25
Radishes, raw, slices (½ cup)	5	13	12	5	10	0.17
Rhubarb, raw, diced (1 cup)	122	10	105	15	17	0.12
Rutabagas, raw, cubes (1 cup)	812	35	66	32	81	0.48
Seaweed						
Agar, dried (100 g)	0	0	625	770	52	5.8
Agar, raw (⅛ cup, 2 tbsp.)	0	0	5	7	1	0.06
Irishmoss, raw (⅛ cup, or 2 tbsp.)	12	0	7	14	16	0.2
Kelp, raw (⅛ cup or 2 tbsp.)	12	0	17	12	4	0.12
Laver, raw (⅛ cup or 2 tbsp.)	520	4	7	0	6	0.11

	VIT A (IU)	VIT C (mg)	CAL (mg)	MAG (mg)	PHOS (mg)	ZINC (mg)
Spirulina, dried (1 cup)	86	2	18	29	18	0.3
Spirulina, raw (1 cup)	56	1	12	19	11	0.2
Wakame, raw (1/8 cup or 2 tbsp.)	36	0	15	11	8	0.04
Shallots, fresh (1 tbsp.)	416	1	4	*	6	*
Spinach						
Cooked, drained (1/2 cup)	7471	9	124	74	51	0.68
Cooked, drained (1 cup)	14,742	18	245	157	101	1.37
Raw (1 cup)	2015	8	30	24	15	0.16
Frozen, chopped or leaf, boiled, drained (1/2 cup)	7395	12	139	66	46	0.67
Frozen, chopped or leaf, boiled, drained (1 cup)	7395	24	278	132	92	1.34
Squash						
Winter, acorn, baked, cubes (1 cup)	877	22	90	88	92	0.35
Winter, acorn, raw, cubes (1/2 cup)	238	9	23	23	25	0.09
Winter, acorn, raw, cubes (1 cup)	476	15	46	45	50	0.18
Winter, butternut, baked (1/2 cup)	7141	15	42	30	28	0.13
Winter, butternut, baked (1 cup)	14,282	31	84	60	55	0.26
Winter, butternut, frozen, boiled, mashed (1/2 cup)	4007	4	23	11	17	0.15
Winter, butternut, frozen, boiled, mashed (1 cup)	8014	8	46	22	34	0.3

	VIT A (IU)	VIT C (mg)	CAL (mg)	MAG (mg)	PHOS (mg)	ZINC (mg)
Winter, spaghetti, boiled or baked, drained, without salt (1/2 cup)	86	3	16	9	11	0.156
Winter, spaghetti, boiled or baked, drained, without salt (1 cup)	162	5	33	17	22	0.312
Zucchini						
Cooked (1/2 cup)	216	4	12	16	36	0.16
Cooked (1 cup)	432	8	24	38	72	0.32
Fresh, baby, raw (1 medium)	54	4	2	4	10	0.09
Frozen, boiled, drained, sliced (1/2 cup)	483	4	19	14	28	0.22
Frozen, boiled, drained, sliced (1 cup)	242	8	38	28	56	0.44
Succotash (corn and limas), boiled, drained (1 cup)	565	16	33	102	225	1.21
Sweet potatoes						
Baked in skin (1 large)	39,280	44	50	36	99	0.52
Boiled, without skin (1 medium)	25,752	26	32	15	41	0.41
Frozen, baked, cubes (1/2 cup)	24,441	8	31	14	34	0.27
Frozen, baked, cubes (1 cup)	28,882	16	62	37	77	0.53
Leaves, steamed, without salt (1/2 cup)	293	0	8	20	19	0.08
Leaves, steamed (1 cup)	586	1	15	39	38	0.17
Raw (1 sweet potato, 5")	26,082	30	29	13	36	0.36

	VIT A (IU)	VIT C (mg)	CAL (mg)	MAG (mg)	PHOS (mg)	ZINC (mg)
Swiss chard, boiled, drained, chopped (1 cup)	5493	32	102	151	58	0.58
Taro, raw, sliced (1 cup)	0	5	45	34	87	0.24
Taro, Tahitian, raw, trimmed, sliced (1/2 cup)	1268	60	80	29	28	*
Taro leaves, steamed (1/2 cup)	3136	26	63	15	20	*
Taro shoots, raw, sliced (1/2 cup)	22	9	5	3	12	*
Tomatillo (1 medium)	39	4	4	13	25	0.15
Tomatillos, raw, chopped (1/2 cup)	75	8	5	13	26	0.15
Tomatoes						
Green, raw (1 medium)	790	29	16	12	34	0.09
Red, ripe, stewed (1 cup)	673	18	26	15	38	0.18
Red, ripe, raw, year-round average (1 medium whole, 1 3/5" dia.)	766	23	6	14	30	0.11
Sun-dried (1 cup)	472	21	59	105	192	1.08
Sun-dried (1 piece)	17	1	2	4	7	0.04
Sun-dried, oil-packed (1 cup)	1415	112	51	90	153	0.86
Sun-dried, oil-packed (1 piece)	39	3	1	2	4	0.02
Turnip, fresh, boiled, drained, mashed (1/2 cup)	0	13	26	9	22	*
Turnip greens, boiled, drained, chopped (1 cup)	7917	40	197	32	42	0.2

	VIT A (IU)	VIT C (mg)	CAL (mg)	MAG (mg)	PHOS (mg)	ZINC (mg)
Turnip greens and turnips, frozen, boiled, drained (100 g)	5161	9	91	12	17	0.13
Water chestnuts, Chinese (matai), raw (1/2 cup)	0	3	7	14	39	0.31
Watercress, raw, chopped (1 cup)	1598	15	41	7	20	0.04
Waxgourd, boiled, drained, cubed (1/2 cup)	0	18	32	*	30	*
Yams, boiled, drained (1/2 cup)	620	8	9	12	33	0.13
Yams, boiled, drained (1 cup)	1240	16	18	24	66	0.26
Yams, mountain, Hawaii, raw (1/2 cup, cubes)	*	1.77	17.9	8.2	23.1	0.16

VEGETABLES, CANNED

	VIT A (IU)	VIT C (mg)	CAL (mg)	MAG (mg)	PHOS (mg)	ZINC (mg)
Asparagus, drained solids (1 cup)	1285	45	39	24	104	0.97
Bamboo shoots, drained solids, slices (1 cup, 1/8")	11	1	11	5	33	0.85
Beans						
Adzuki, mature seeds, sweetened (1/2 cup)	8	0	33	46	110	2.31
Adzuki, mature seeds, sweetened (1 cup)	15	0	65	92	219	4.62
Baked, plain or vegetarian (1/2 cup)	144	*	57	37	118	1.56

	VIT A (IU)	VIT C (mg)	CAL (mg)	MAG (mg)	PHOS (mg)	ZINC (mg)
Baked, plain or vegetarian (1 cup)	388	*	114	73	236	3.17
Black, with liquid (1/2 cup)	5	3	42	42	130	0.65
Black, with liquid (1 cup)	10	6	84	84	269	1.3
Broad (fava), mature seeds (1/2 cup)	13	3	34	41	101	0.8
Broad (fava), mature seeds (1 cup)	26	5	67	82	202	1.59
Chickpeas (garbanzos, bengal gram), mature seeds (1/2 cup)	29	5	39	35	108	1.27
Chickpeas (garbanzos, bengal gram), mature seeds (1 cup)	58	9	77	70	216	2.54
Cranberry (Roman), mature seed (1/2 cup)	0	1	44	42	112	1.09
Cranberry (Roman), mature seed (1 cup)	0	2	88	83	224	2.18
Great Northern, mature seeds (1/2 cup)	2	2	70	67	178	0.85
Great Northern, mature seeds (1 cup)	3	3	139	134	356	1.7
Hyacinth, cooked (1/2 cup)	44	5	20	18	22	*
Hyacinth, raw (1 cup)	88	10	40	36	44	*
Green, drained (1/2 cup)	300	4	18	9	13	0.2

	VIT A (IU)	VIT C (mg)	CAL (mg)	MAG (mg)	PHOS (mg)	ZINC (mg)
Green, drained (1 cup)	599	7	36	18	26	0.4
Italian, green/yellow (1/2 cup)	80	2	18	9	*	*
Italian, green/yellow (1 cup)	159	4	35	18	*	*
Kidney, all types, mature seeds (1/2 cup)	0	2	35	40	135	0.7
Kidney, all types, mature seeds (1 cup)	0	3	69	79	269	1.41
Kidney, red, mature seeds (1/2 cup)	0	2	31	36	121	0.7
Kidney, red, mature seeds (1 cup)	0	3	61	72	241	1.41
Lima, large, mature seeds (1/2 cup)	0	0	26	47	89	0.79
Lima, large, mature seeds (1 cup)	0	0	51	94	178	1.57
Mung, mature seeds sprouted, drained solids (1/2 cup)	15	0	9	6	20	0.18
Mung, mature seeds sprouted, drained solids (1 cup)	29	0	18	11	40	0.35
Navy, mature seeds (1/2 cup)	2	1	62	62	176	1.01
Navy, mature seeds (1 cup)	3	2	123	123	351	2.02
Pigeonpeas, boiled, drained (1/2 cup)	100	22	32	*	32	0.63
Pigeonpeas, boiled, drained (1 cup)	200	43	63	*	63	1.26
Pinto, mature seeds (1/2 cup)	2	1	52	33	111	0.83
Pinto, mature seeds (1 cup)	58	2	103	65	221	1.66

	VIT A (IU)	VIT C (mg)	CAL (mg)	MAG (mg)	PHOS (mg)	ZINC (mg)
Refried, fat-free (1/2 cup)	0	8	45	42	108	1.47
Refried, fat-free (1 cup)	0	16	90	84	216	0.74
Refried, vegetarian (1/2 cup)	500	6	40	*	*	*
Refried, vegetarian (1 cup)	1000	12	80	*	*	*
Shell, solids and liquids (1/2 cup)	280	4	36	19	37	0.33
Shell, solids and liquids (1 cup)	559	8	71	37	74	0.66
Snap, green, regular pack, drained solids (1/2 cup)	236	4	18	9	13	0.2
Snap, green, regular pack, drained solids (1 cup)	471	7	35	18	26	0.39
Snap, yellow, regular pack, drained, solids (1/2 cup)	71	3.5	18	9	13	0.2
Snap, yellow, regular pack, drained, solids (1 cup)	142	7	35	18	26	0.39
White, mature seeds (1/2 cup)	0	0	96	67	119	1.47
White, mature seeds (1 cup)	0	0	191	134	238	2.93
Bean sprouts (1 cup)	8	30	11	36	*	*
Beets						
Drained solids, slices (1/2 cup)	10	4	13	15	15	0.18
Drained solids, slices (1 cup)	19	7	26	29	29	0.36
Harvard, solids and liquids, slices (1/2 cup)	14	3	14	24	21	0.29

	VIT A (IU)	VIT C (mg)	CAL (mg)	MAG (mg)	PHOS (mg)	ZINC (mg)
Harvard, solids and liquids, slices (1 cup)	27	6	27	47	42	0.57
Pickled, solids and liquids, slices (1/2 cup)	13	3	13	17	20	0.3
Pickled, solids and liquids, slices (1 cup)	25	5	25	34	39	0.59
Carrots, regular pack, drained solids (1/2 cup)	10,055	2	19	6	18	0.19
Carrots, regular pack, drained solids (1 cup)	20,110	4	37	12	35	0 38
Corn						
Red and green peppers, solids and liquids (1/2 cup)	264	10	6	29	71	0.12
Red and green peppers, solids and liquids (1 cup)	527	20	11	57	141	0.64
White, sweet, cream-style, regular pack (1/2 cup)	0	6	4	22	66	0.68
White, sweet, cream-style, regular pack (1 cup)	0	12	8	44	131	1.36
Yellow, sweet, cream-style, regular pack (1/2 cup)	124	6	4	22	66	0.68
Yellow, sweet, cream-style, regular pack (1 cup)	248	12	8	44	131	1.36

	VIT A (IU)	VIT C (mg)	CAL (mg)	MAG (mg)	PHOS (mg)	ZINC (mg)
Yellow, sweet, cream-style, special dietary pack (1/2 cup)	124	6	4	22	66	0.68
Yellow, sweet, cream-style, special dietary pack (1 cup)	248	12	8	44	131	1.36
Yellow, sweet, whole kernel, drained solids (1/2 cup)	128	7	4	17	54	0.32
Yellow, sweet, whole kernel, drained solids (1 cup)	256	14	8	33	107	0.64
Cowpeas, common (black-eyed crowder, Southern), mature seeds plain (1/2 cup)	16	4	24	34	84	0.84
Cowpeas, common (black-eyed crowder, Southern), mature seeds plain (1 cup)	31	7	48	67	168	1.68
Hominy, white (1/2 cup)	0	0	8.5	23	29	0.87
Hominy, white (1 cup)	0	0	17	26	58	1.73
Hominy, yellow (1/2 cup)	88	0	8	23	28	0.84
Hominy, yellow (1 cup)	176	0	16	26	56	1.68
Hearts of palm (1 piece)	0	3	19	13	22	0.38
Mushrooms, drained solids (1/2 cup)	0	0	9	12	52	0.56
Mushrooms, drained solids (1 cup)	0	0	18	24	104	1.12
Olives, ripe (1 large)	18	0	4	0	0	0.01
Olives, ripe (10 large)	180	0	40	0	0	0.1
Peas, green, regular pack, drained solids (1/2 cup)	653	8	17	15	57	0.61

	VIT A (IU)	VIT C (mg)	CAL (mg)	MAG (mg)	PHOS (mg)	ZINC (mg)
Peas, green, regular pack, drained solids (1 cup)	1306	16	34	29	114	1.21
Peas, seasoned, with liquid (1/2 cup)	494	13	18	17	61	0.74
Peas, seasoned, with liquid (1 cup)	988	26	36	34	122	1.48
Peas and carrots, regular pack, solids and liquids (1/2 cup)	7357	9	30	18	59	0.74
Peas and carrots, regular pack, solids and liquids (1 cup)	14,714	17	59	36	117	1.48
Peas and onions, solid and liquids (1/2 cup)	97	2	10	10	31	0.04
Peas and onions, solid and liquids (1 cup)	193	4	20	19	61	0.7
Peppers						
Hot chili, green, pods, chopped, diced (1/2 cup)	415	46	5	10	12	0.12
Hot chili, green, pods, chopped, diced (1 cup)	830	92	10	20	24	0.24
Jalapeño, solids and liquids (1/2 cup chopped)	1156	9	18	8	12	0.13
Jalapeño, solids and liquids (1 cup chopped)	2312	18	35	16	23	0.26
Jute, potherb, raw (1/2 cup)	778	5	58	32	23	0.22
Jute, potherb, raw (1 cup)	1556	10	58	32	23	0.22
Sweet, green, solids and liquids, halves (1/2 cup)	109	33	29	8	24	0.13

	VIT A (IU)	VIT C (mg)	CAL (mg)	MAG (mg)	PHOS (mg)	ZINC (mg)
Sweet, green, solids and liquids, halves (1 cup)	217	65	57	15	28	0.25
Pimento (1 whole)	1752	56	4	4	11	0.13
Potatoes, drained solids (1/2 cup)	0	5	5	13	35	0.25
Potatoes, drained solids (1 cup)	0	10	9	25	50	0.5
Pumpkin (1/2 cup)	26,908	5	32	28	42	0.21
Pumpkin (1 cup)	53,816	10	64	56	84	0.42
Pumpkin pie mix (1/2 cup)	11,202	5	50	22	61	0.37
Pumpkin pie mix (1 cup)	22,405	10	100	43	122	0.73
Sauerkraut, solids and liquids (1/2 cup)	13	11	22	10	24	0.14
Sauerkraut, solids and liquids (1 cup)	26	21	43	19	28	0.27
Spinach, drained solids (1/2 cup)	9391	16	136	82	47	0.49
Spinach, drained solids (1 cup)	18,781	31	272	163	94	0.98
Spinach, New Zealand, raw (1/2 cup)	1232	8	16	11	9	0.11
Spinach, New Zealand, raw (1 cup)	2464	17	32	22	18	0.21
Squash, summer, crookneck, straightneck, drained solid, slices (1/2 cup)	131	3	13	14	23	0.32
Squash, summer, crookneck, straightneck, drained solid, slices (1 cup)	261	6	26	28	45	0.63
Squash, summer zucchini, Italian-style (1/2 cup)	612	3	20	16	33	0.30

	VIT A (IU)	VIT C (mg)	CAL (mg)	MAG (mg)	PHOS (mg)	ZINC (mg)
Squash, summer zucchini, Italian-style (1 cup)	1224	5	39	32	66	0.59
Succotash (corn and limas) with cream-style corn (1/2 cup)	187.5	9	15	2	79	0.57
Succotash (corn and limas) with cream-style corn (1 cup)	375	17	29	3	157	1.14
Sweet potato, syrup pack, drained, solids (1/2 cup)	7014	11	17	12	25	0.15
Sweet potato, syrup pack, drained, solids (1 cup)	14,028	21	33	24	49	0.31
Sweet potato, vacuum pack, pieces (1/2 cup)	7988	27	22	22	49	0.18
Sweet potato, vacuum pack, pieces (1 cup)	15,966	53	44	44	98	0.36
Tomato products						
Paste, without salt added (1 tbsp.)	4001	7	6	8	13	0.13
Puree, with salt added (1 cup)	3188	26	43	60	100	0.55
Red, ripe, stewed (1 cup)	1380	29	84	31	51	0.43
Red, ripe, wedges in tomato juice (1 cup)	1509	39	68	29	60	0.42
Red, ripe, with green chilies (1 cup)	940	15	48	27	34	0.31
Sauce, with mushrooms (1 cup)	2340	30	32	47	78	0.51
Sauce, with onions (1 cup)	2083	31	42	47	96	0.56

	VIT A (IU)	VIT C (mg)	CAL (mg)	MAG (mg)	PHOS (mg)	ZINC (mg)
Sauce, with tomato tidbits (1 cup)	1954	53	24	49	103	0.46
Turnip greens, solids and liquids (1/2 cup)	4196	18	138	23	25	0.27
Turnip greens, solids and liquids (1 cup)	8292	36	276	46	50	0.54
Vegetables, mixed, drained solids (1/2 cup)	9493	4	22	13	35	0.34
Vegetables, mixed, drained solids (1 cup)	18,985	8	44	26	69	0.67
Water chestnuts, Chinese, solids and liquds (1/2 cup)	3	1	3	4	13	0.27
Water chestnuts, Chinese, solids and liquids (1 cup)	6	2	6	8	26	0.54

21-DAY BONE-BOOSTING DIARY

Fill in the amount of foods or beverages eaten each day along with the key bone-boosting nutrients. A sample has been given to assist you. Check with the **Bone-Boosting Requirements (BBR)** listed on page 18 to make sure you are getting ample vitamins and minerals to keep bones strong and prevent osteoporosis.

21-DAY BONE-BOOSTING DIARY

	Food/Beverage	Amount	BBR Nutrients
Day 1	milk	8 ounces	cal, vit D, phos, vit A, mag
	scrambled eggs	2 whole eggs	phos, vit A
	orange	1 small	vit C, vit A
	whole wheat toast	2 pieces	cal, phos, mag

	Food/Beverage
Day 1	

Amount	BBR Nutrients

	Food/Beverage
Day 2	

Amount	BBR Nutrients

	Food/Beverage
Day 3	

Amount	BBR Nutrients

	Food/Beverage
Day 4	

Amount	BBR Nutrients

	Food/Beverage
Day 5	

Amount	BBR Nutrients

	Food/Beverage
Day 6	

Amount	BBR Nutrients

	Food/Beverage
Day 7	

Amount	BBR Nutrients

	Food/Beverage
Day 8	

Amount	BBR Nutrients

	Food/Beverage
Day 9	

Amount	BBR Nutrients

	Food/Beverage
Day 10	

Amount	BBR Nutrients

	Food/Beverage
Day 11	

Amount	BBR Nutrients

	Food/Beverage
Day 12	

Amount	BBR Nutrients

	Food/Beverage
Day 13	

Amount	BBR Nutrients

	Food/Beverage
Day 14	

Amount	BBR Nutrients

	Food/Beverage
Day 15	

Amount	BBR Nutrients

	Food/Beverage
Day 16	

Amount	BBR Nutrients

	Food/Beverage
Day 17	

Amount	BBR Nutrients

	Food/Beverage
Day 18	

Amount	BBR Nutrients

	Food/Beverage
Day 19	

Amount	BBR Nutrients

	Food/Beverage
Day 20	

Amount	BBR Nutrients

	Food/Beverage
Day 21	

Amount	BBR Nutrients

EAT HEALTHY WITH KENSINGTON